The Everyman's Guide to Hair Replacement

The Everyman's Guide to Hair Replacement

Richard W. Fleming, M.D., F.A.C.S.
Clinical Professor, Otolaryngology-Head and Neck Surgery
Division of Facial Plastic and Reconstructive Surgery
University of Southern California
Los Angeles, California

Toby G. Mayer, M.D., F.A.C.S.
Clinical Professor, Otolaryngology-Head and Neck Surgery
Division of Facial Plastic and Reconstructive Surgery
University of Southern California
Los Angeles, California

EquiMedia Corporation
Austin • Yokohama

Authors	Richard W. Fleming, M.D., F.A.C.S.
	Toby G. Mayer, M.D., F.A.C.S.
Editor	Perry Luckett
Art Director/Design	Robert Feinberg
Illustrator	Timothy C. Hengst
Production Assistant	Taro Kodama
Research Assistant	Irene Luckett
Hair Additions Consultant	Michael Mahoney
Hair Styling	Adamo Lentini
Cover Photography	Andy Pearlman Studio

Library of Congress Cataloging-in-Publication Data
Fleming, Richard W.
    The everyman's guide to hair replacement / Richard W. Fleming,
Toby G. Mayer. -- 1st ed.
        p. cm.
    Includes bibliographical references and index.
    ISBN 0-9625898-1-0 (pbk.) : $14.95. -- ISBN 0-9625898-2-9 : $19.95
    1. Baldness--Popular works.   I. Mayer, Toby G.   II. Title.
RL155.F54 1994
616.5'46--dc20   94-18092
                                                        CIP

Published by
EquiMedia Corporation
P.O. Box 90519
Austin, Texas 78709
512-288-1676

Printed in Singapore

Contents

Preface 7

Introduction 9

Chapter 1.   Hair Structure and Growth 11

Chapter 2.   Temporary Hair Loss 15

Chapter 3.   Permanent Hair Loss (Baldness) 23

Chapter 4.   Styling for Best Appearance 29

Chapter 5.   Non-surgical Hair Additions 43

Chapter 6.   Other Non-surgical Approaches 67

Chapter 7.   Prescription Drugs Under Development ... 79

Chapter 8.   Scalp Reductions 89

Chapter 9.   Transplants 101

Chapter 10.   Flap Surgery 121

Chapter 11.   The Forehead Lift 141

Chapter 12.   Tissue Expansion 149

Chapter 13.   Other Flaps Used for Scalp Surgery 157

Chapter 14.   Reconstructive Surgery 163

Chapter 15.   Choosing a Doctor 173

Glossary 179
Bibliography 187
Index 189
Credits 192

Preface

If you're concerned about your hair loss, you're not alone. A recent study by Dr. Thomas Cash, Professor of Psychology at Old Dominion University, shows that balding men are very sensitive about their condition. Nearly 84 percent wish for more hair. More than two-thirds spend time looking in the mirror at their hair and wonder what others think of them. Almost 80 percent get teased by their peers about their baldness and, although they might laugh along with friends, inside they're not laughing. Instead, they feel self-conscious and helpless. Many men even feel that their hair is a symbol of their virility and youth, so their self-esteem drops a bit with each falling strand.

Unfortunately, society's perceptions about baldness have helped create these negative feelings. Another study by Dr. Cash used 18 pairs of balding and nonbalding men's photographs to see how people would view them in terms of various social characteristics. The men were matched by age and race, and they approved the photographs as either representing or improving their actual appearance.

An equal number of men and women viewed these photographs in random order, with startling results. They consistently saw bald or balding men as less physically attractive, less assertive, less socially attractive, less likely to be successful in their personal and social lives, and less likeable. They also thought balding or bald men were five years older, on average, than their nonbalding counterparts. Small wonder, then, that balding men worry about their hair loss.

These anxieties and perceptions concerning baldness have been with us throughout recorded history. Nearly 3,500 years ago, balding Egyptians were seeking a "cure" that required a poultice of equal parts of the fats from the ibex, lion, crocodile, serpent, goose, and hippopotamus together with the burned prickles of a hedgehog immersed in oil, fingernail scrapings, and a mix of honey, alabaster, and red ochre. Obviously, the Egyptians were concerned enough about hair loss to take some significant risks in trying to solve it.

Today's solutions for baldness may appear more scientific and easier to accept, but they otherwise drive at the same basic need: to get back the hairline we used to enjoy seeing in the mirror. If you've lost some or most of your hair, you've probably at least begun the frustrating process of trying to deal with your loss. Perhaps you've struggled with combing and recombing your hair to cover thinning spots. You've tried special shampoos and conditioners which promise to "deep clean" your hair follicles and promote healthy growth. Or you've gone on special diets and taken nutritional supplements to give your hair back the nutrients it appears to be missing. You may even have repeatedly (and futilely) massaged your scalp or rubbed quantities of exotic lotions on your head to coax back what has disappeared with alarming swiftness. These and other treatments have become part of a multi-billion dollar business in hair restoration.

Whether you're just beginning your journey toward restoration or are already a weary traveler, this book will guide you on the road to an educated decision about your hair loss. It is an objective doctor's view of which hair-replacement methods work and which ones don't, designed so you can choose areas that interest you and quickly find key facts about them. We hope this book will clear up a lot of misinformation while saving you considerable money and disappointment.

In the following pages, you'll discover all of the approaches to treating baldness, along with the products or techniques associated with them. You'll find clear information on hair growth and loss, as well as styling your remaining hair for best coverage. You'll also read the latest news about lotions, creams, injections, diets, electrical stimulation, weaves, hairpieces, transplants, and recent surgical techniques for hair replacement.

Because the authors have more than 20 years of experience treating thousands of patients with all surgical methods of hair replacement, they can discuss all of these techniques objectively and in plain terms, yet thoroughly enough so you'll understand each procedure. They also summarize the disadvantages, advantages, and costs of these methods, so you'll find it easy to compare them. Charts and illustrations explain key ideas in clear form. And "before and after" photographs often allow you to see the results for yourself.

The key to choosing properly from the options available to you is to be fully informed about all of them. We want you to know enough about every possibility so you can make up your mind whether to "live with" your loss or to take a reasonable course toward solving it. As you'll see, we've come a long way since balding Egyptians thought they had to wrestle lions and crocodiles in order to take off their headdresses in public!

I should know. I've experienced not only the anxiety of losing my hair but also the waste of time and money spent chasing false hopes and promises of a head of hair that would be just like it used to be.

After years of disappointment upon disappointment, my personal journey ended with the discovery of the Fleming/Mayer Flap. How do I look? That's me on the cover.

Robert Feinberg
President
Equimedia Publishing, Inc.

Introduction

Throughout recorded history, there has always been an intense interest in hair and its social significance. Hairstyles were used as a method of class distinction in ancient cultures. Many superstitions about hair include its correlation with physical strength, magical rites, and folklore. For centuries, society has had a negative attitude about baldness. Many forms of ancient treatment have been recorded. Mixtures of animal parts, snakes, and vegetable material including roots, oils, brans and flowers have been prescribed. Archaeologists have discovered wigs thousands of years old.

There still is a pervasive belief that baldness is not desirable. Many men experience significant psychological trauma with the loss of their hair. Having grown up with a face framed by hair, they experience a tremendous adjustment in their self image with this loss.

This book is not humorous, full of anecdotal stories about glorifying hair loss. Few agree that "bald is beautiful." Most people who experience baldness, a condition which they cannot control, don't want to be entertained; they want facts about reasonable treatments. Very few men would have a bald scalp if they clearly understood the sensible alternatives. Unethical opportunists take advantage of these vulnerable individuals promoting ineffective and inappropriate hair growth products and surgical procedures.

We have written this book, sharing over 20 years of experience in the treatment of baldness, because there is a need for accurate information. Misconceptions about the treatment of baldness are rampant. Most men do not share their feelings about hair loss or any treatment they had for this condition. Although we have many patients who are celebrities and public figures, they are very private about their experiences. There are alternative approaches depending on the type of hair, extent of baldness and personal desires. We discuss the causes of hair loss, hairstyling, medical treatments, hair additions (hairpieces), and surgical alternatives.

The media is fascinated with medical "cures." However, the FDA has not approved any "across the counter" preparations and only one prescription drug for the treatment of hair loss. Medical treatments are discussed in detail.

Hair additions are an excellent alternative for some individuals. Various types of products and methods of attachment are described.

We chronicle the evolution of hair replacement surgery over the past 30 years, emphasizing the advantages and disadvantages of each procedure. In our practice, we use all techniques, not promoting a single procedure. We provide an overview of hair replacement surgery with an emphasis on the Fleming-Mayer Flap, which we feel is best for most individuals.

Initially, we used only the circular punch grafts, popularly know as hair transplants, which was the only technique available at that time. Unfortunately a tufted, "picket fence" appearance was always present after the work was completed. The process was slow, taking two to three years to achieve the final result. New methods of punch grafting include smaller micrografts and minigrafts which have only two to five hairs in each graft. Therefore, the tufting and row-of-corn appearance is less of a problem. We use this approach on some individuals but normal density can never be achieved.

Flaps were a significant advancement in the treatment of baldness. They provided immediate results with hair of normal uniform density. In a man with only frontal baldness, it is eliminated in two weeks. Popularized by Dr. J. Juri in 1975, we have made many changes in the technique and, therefore, the evolution of the Fleming-Mayer Flap.

Other significant developments include scalp reductions, used in conjunction with hair transplants and flap surgery. With this operation, we remove some bald skin and then stretch the surrounding hair-bearing scalp to close the resulting defect.

The use of tissue expanders to stretch normal hair-bearing skin is an exciting, valuable technique for use in both reconstructive surgery and the treatment of male-pattern baldness. This procedure, which is described in detail, gives us the opportunity to decrease or eliminate baldness that previously was beyond surgical repair.

These techniques are described in detail. Every patient should consider all options. During the selection process, remember the axiom "baldness is progressive." Most who experience hair loss will have baldness over the entire top of the head. The greatest source of a patient disappointment is not having a clear understanding of the anticipated result. Before selecting a particular technique, always see an individual with similar type of hair and extent of baldness whose hair replacement is complete.

Hopefully this book will be the first step in the process of understanding your hair loss, considering all reasonable options, and finally selecting the approach that will satisfy your expectations.

1.
Hair Structure
& Growth

Hair growth in humans is truly remarkable because each hair follicle has its own "program" that controls how long a hair will grow, as well as when it will fall out and be replaced by another growing hair. Hair grows at different rates and in varying patterns, textures, and thicknesses, depending on its purpose and location on your body. Because this book focuses on hair replacement, however, we'll concentrate on the hair covering the human scalp. Knowing more about the nature of hair—including its structure, types, and growth phases—will prepare you for later discussions on hair loss.

The hair on your head grows about one-half inch per month from follicles in the scalp. These "stocking-like" follicles are surrounded by a very dense system of blood vessels that provide the oxygen and nutrients your hair needs to grow (fig. 1-1). At the base of each follicle is an area of closely connected tissue—called the papilla—which folds over the lower ends of the hairs. Each hair rests in a sheath which contains keratin (a protein) and the grains of melanin that determine your hair color.

In healthy follicles, the cells lying over the hair papilla form, divide, absorb protein in the form of keratin, and then lose moisture and die. Eventually, they build up a lace of dead cells cemented together by amino acid.

This mass of "keratinized" cells makes up the hair shaft. When new cells form at the base of the follicle, they push the shaft up and out, and your hair grows. Thus, your hair is nothing more than dead cells united in the form of keratin (protein) threads.

Hair has three distinct layers (fig. 1-2). The "cuticle," or outside layer, has flat, transparent cells that overlap each other like shingles or fish scales. They protect the inside of the hair shaft. When stylists talk about damaged hair, they're usually referring to this outer layer, which can be torn by rough combs or brushes and broken down by chemicals.

The second layer is the "cortex"—made up of oblong cells that grow end to end rather than overlap. The cortex gives your hair shape, flexibility, and natural color. The inside layer of your hair, or "medulla," contains two rows of cells that grow side by side over the length of the shaft. The medulla determines each hair's strength, body, and elasticity.

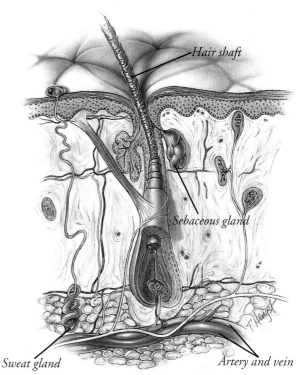

Fig. 1-1. Section of hair follicle in the skin surrounded by blood vessels (arteries and veins) and sebaceous glands.

Individual hairs stay soft, shiny, and pliable because nearby sebaceous glands secrete an oily material (sebum) into the hair follicle near the surface of the skin (fig. 1-1). This sebum lubricates the hair fiber and reduces friction. Overproduction or underproduction of sebum causes oily or dry hair, respectively. In some cases, too much sebum can even cause a balding condition called Alopecia Seborrheica—a temporary problem that has nothing to do with male pattern baldness.

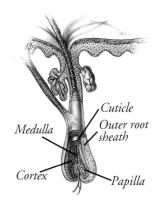

Fig. 1-2. Three layers of hair (cuticle, cortex, and medulla) within it's follicle.

Human scalp hair is remarkable for its potential length (40 inches or more), its strength, and its ability to stretch up to 30 percent before breaking. It comes in two forms: vellus and terminal. Vellus hair is soft, short, and usually uncolored. It's the kind of hair that often grows on bald scalps, giving them a "peach fuzz" appearance. Terminal hair is long, more brittle, and colored. It is the "normal" hair that gives us our hairline and style, so it's an important part of our self image.

If you're a brown- or black-haired person with normal hair, you have about 100,000 terminal hairs in your scalp. That compares to 140,000 if you're a blond and 90,000 if you're a redhead. These numbers may surprise you because brunettes look like they have more hair than blonds. That's because a brunette's hair is coarser in texture, which gives it more "body." Red hair compensates for its relative scarceness by being thicker, heavier, and usually coarser than all other hair colors.

The Hair Growth Cycle

All hair goes through three phases: growth (anagen), transition (catagen), and rest (telogen). Typically, about 90 percent of your hairs are growing and about 10 percent are resting or shedding. That's why, if you have a normal head of hair, you can expect up to 100 hairs a day to fall out onto your hairbrush, comb, pillow, or shower drain. In other words, this amount of shedding is perfectly natural and is no cause for alarm.

Your hair's growing phase, or anagen, lasts two to five years. Hair can grow to 40 inches or more, but at the end of this period it enters a transitional phase, called catagen. This transitional phase lasts about two or three weeks. Although your hair is still long and visible during catagen, it's no longer growing. Below the scalp's surface the hair follicle shrinks and becomes dormant. A small bulb of keratin appears at the base of the hair and causes the lower end of the hair to take on a club-like shape. The keratin also holds the hair weakly in place within the follicle until telogen begins (fig. 1-3).

Certain common events alter the shedding of hair. For example, during pregnancy more follicles are maintained in the growing phase, so there is less shedding than usual. About three months after delivery, some 30 percent of the follicles simultaneously enter the resting phase, causing a heavy loss of hair that is temporary and self-correcting.

Understanding the hair growth cycle and its variations helps us realize that some temporary shedding is normal. As long as your hair continues to be replaced by new growth, you need not be concerned. In some cases, though, hair may fall out and not be replaced after the usual resting phase. As you'll see in the next two chapters, we must determine whether this type of loss will be temporary or permanent before deciding how to treat it.

Fig. 1-3. During telogen, or the resting phase, the dormant hair works its way out of the follicle and falls out. Meantime, over the next three to four months, a new hair is forming and growing toward the surface of your scalp. This new hair will follow the same cycle: growth for two to five years, shedding, and resting.

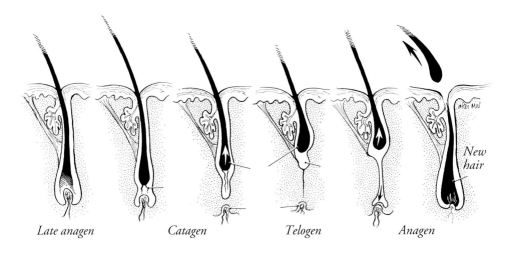

Late anagen   Catagen   Telogen   Anagen

New hair

2.
Temporary Hair Loss

Because hair depends on healthy cells and nutrients in the hair follicles, certain conditions, diseases, or drugs can temporarily interrupt the growth cycle. When new hairs don't form after the resting phase, the scalp takes on a thinning or bald appearance. Although this type of loss can be traumatic, hair usually grows normally once the cause is removed. In this chapter, we'll introduce you to the most common causes of temporary hair loss. However, because they are often complex, you should consult a doctor if you have any of these conditions.

Alopecia Areata

Translated, this phrase means patchy baldness, a condition that appears suddenly in people who have no apparent skin disorder or disease. Both men and women experience it--at the rate of less than one in a thousand, usually in the younger age groups (ages 20-40). Heavy or early hair loss may cause permanent baldness, but more than 60 percent of people with alopecia areata have at least partial regrowth within a year. Unfortunately, about 70-80 percent suffer one or more additional episodes of this disease.

If you have alopecia areata, your barber or hairdresser may be the first to notice it because you'll have no other symptoms. You can identify it by a white, roundish or oval patch with smooth, curved edges and

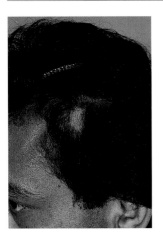 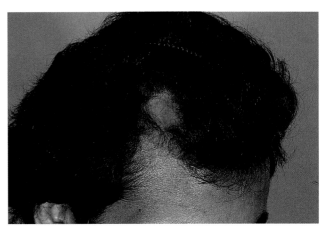

Fig. 2-1a (above) and Fig. 2-1b (above right). Patient has round patchy areas of baldness because of alopecia areata.

short stubble hair on the surface (fig. 2-1). Often, easily plucked hairs grow around the edge of the patch. They're shaped like exclamation points and result only from this kind of baldness or from anti-cancer drugs.

Patchy baldness is largely untreatable because we still don't know what causes it. Hints about connections to the immune system or to heredity aren't conclusive. Treatments of symptoms with various steroids, caustic agents, or radiation have had limited success. Sometimes, local injections of cortisone have helped regrow hair in very specific areas, such as the eyebrows.

Because doctors can't predict how (and how often) this kind of baldness will occur, they usually can't use scalp reduction or transplant surgery to cover it. In certain cases, when the condition has been stable for some time, hair replacement surgery may be possible. Surgeons can't guarantee that baldness won't recur, but chances are excellent that the results will be good. If surgery isn't possible, you must wait for your hair to regrow, wear something on your head (a hair addition, hat, cap, or scarf), or shave your scalp. Unfortunately, if you have alopecia areata, chasing nonexistent cures will only cost you time and money.

Drugs

The most widely known cause of hair loss associated with medical treatment is chemotherapy to combat cancer. All anti-cancer medications are toxic to your body's cells. They stop the cell division and growth that normally goes on in the hair bulb, so hair growth can't continue. Thus, if you must take such anticancer drugs as methotrexate, adriamycin, vinblastine, or busulfan--to name a few, you can expect temporary hair loss over up to 90 percent of your scalp.

Many other drugs have been known to cause temporary baldness, although some are connected to only one or a few cases. Several researchers have written about these drugs, which include amphetamines, birth-control pills, medicines that fight inflammation or thin the blood, anabolic steroids, male hormones (testosterone or androgens), and many others. Discontinuing oral contraceptives or taking too much vitamin A can also cause hair loss. Unfortunately, you need to be prepared for undesirable side effects when you take needed prescription medicines or overdo certain dietary supplements.

Dandruff, Seborrhea, Psoriasis

Dandruff appears to result from a slight increase in the normal 28-day turnover of skin, causing the excess to scale off in white flakes. Seborrhea comes from inflamed sebaceous (oil) glands, which redden the scalp and produce scales thicker and more plentiful than those from dandruff. Psoriasis also develops from an inflamed scalp. Because this inflamed skin turns over ten times faster than normal, psoriasis may create large amounts of scaling and some swelling on patches of skin.

If you're losing hair from any of these conditions, take heart--it's only temporary and reversible. Often, rubbing and scratching will break hairs and force them out. Because the causes of scaling aren't entirely clear, your best bet is care rather than cure. Avoid buildup of hair sprays and gels. Increase frequency of shampooing and make sure your conditioner is right for your hair type. If you're still troubled by scaliness, try a "therapeutic shampoo"--usually containing sulfur-salicylic acid, tar, zinc pyrithione, or selenium sulfide. Of course, you should stop using any product that irritates your scalp. And consult a doctor if your condition continues.

Poor Nutrition

Most cases of hair thinning from nutritional problems occur in underdeveloped countries which have food supplies near starvation levels. But abnormal eating habits, such as crash or fad diets, can also cause hair to thin. Crash diets have too few daily calories, and fad diets often exclude essential foods. If you lack protein, carbohydrates, fats, or certain vitamins, your hair's health will be affected.

Because your hair is mostly protein (keratin), it needs protein to stay healthy. Too little of this nutrient can lead to a temporary loss of color and texture. The resulting thin, dry hair sheds easily. A protein deficiency can also cause more of your hairs to go into telogen and, if not corrected in time, develop permanent baldness.

Carbohydrates and fats contribute to the normal activities of growing hair, so you shouldn't try to eliminate either from your diet. Carbohydrates provide energy that helps your body use protein and improve cell growth in your hair follicles. Fats are important to the sebaceous glands, which produce the sebum that naturally conditions your hair. In fact, sebum itself is a fat, specially composed to keep the hair follicles lubricated.

Although deficiencies in vitamin B complex and vitamin C can cause problems for your hair and scalp, vitamin A is most important to healthy hair. As we've pointed out, you must be careful not to take in too much vitamin A. But if you take in too little of this vitamin, your hair may become dry and dull. Eventually, you may even lose hair because hair bulbs die or form cysts when they don't get enough vitamin A.

Researchers have shown that a vitamin A deficiency can cause the outer layer of your scalp skin to grow over the mouths of your hair follicles near the sebaceous glands. This growth then obstructs the openings of the follicles, slows hair development, and keeps sebum from flowing properly. Because the keratin cells continue growing, they may form "plugs" that block the hair from coming out and cause the sebaceous glands to wither. Hair loss is the result.

Certain illnesses can also lead to poor nutrition and partial baldness. If you were suffering from severe problems of the gastrointestinal tract, for example, your inability to keep food down could cause this kind of malnutrition. If a prolonged stay in a hospital required you to be on intravenous feeding--or if you otherwise didn't get enough fatty acid, biotin, and zinc--you could lose scalp hair.

Trauma from Pulling or Pressure

A common cause of temporary hair loss is "traction alopecia," which can develop if you use devices to hold, straighten, or curl your hair. Typical examples are curlers, pins, ponytail ties, tight barrettes, picks for curly or kinky hair, and nylon brushes. You may also cause this problem by pulling your hair into popular styles: pigtails, ponytails, braids, or cornrows. Removing the traction normally allows your hair to regrow. But if you use these devices or styles continuously, your hair follicles will develop permanent scars — leading to permanent hair loss (fig. 2-2).

Another self-induced type of hair loss stems from "trichotillomania"--a neurotic compulsion to pull the hair. For the most part, it occurs only in children and teenagers, often because of emotional disturbances, such as dissatisfaction with body image or a family conflict. Psychological or psychiatric evaluation typically leads to a solution.

You could also lose hair if you had to lie in one position for a long time--perhaps because of an extended surgery, coma, or other illness that kept you from moving on your own. Doctors call this hair loss "pressure alopecia" and believe it probably results from poor

Fig. 2-2. Hair loss caused by attaching a hairpiece. If traction on hair is tight and continuous, permanent scarring and hair loss can result.

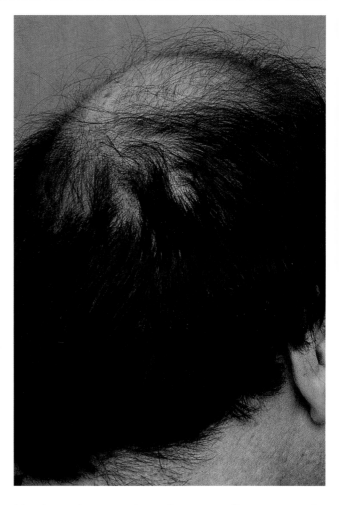

blood circulation in the scalp. It usually continues for up to a month after the event that causes it. Relieving the pressure allows normal scalp circulation, so attendants can turn or move a patient more frequently to help prevent this kind of baldness.

Infection, Disease, and Other Stress

In the early 1960s, doctors observed hair loss from stress and identified it as "telogen effluvium"--an abrupt interruption of the growth phase followed by shedding. If you have an emotional disturbance, a prolonged fever, certain diseases, or surgery, up to three times the normal number of your hair follicles may go prematurely into telogen. About two to four months after the stressful event, new hair buds would push your telogen hairs out, causing heavy and diffuse shedding of normal club hairs. Once the cause of this condition disappears, unless the stress is very great, your hair would regrow completely within six months.

An infection is one disorder that could attack your hair follicles or otherwise indirectly cause this kind of hair loss. Although doctors aren't certain of the relationship between infection and telogen effluvium in all cases, they do know that the fungi which infect hair follicles keep hair from growing properly. For example, tumors in follicles cause hair loss, and when syphilis infects the body, it causes a characteristic "moth-eaten" or scaly scalp.

Diseases that affect your metabolism (chemical changes in the cells) can also lead to baldness. For example, diabetics whose condition isn't controlled often lose hair over much of their scalps. Poor circulation to the scalp, a lack of insulin, or toxic effects from changes in the way their bodies handle carbohydrates and fats are all possible causes of this loss.

Another common metabolic disease that produces some hair loss is hypothyroidism--when the thyroid gland puts out too little hormone. Malfunction in the gland, heavy use of antithyroid drugs, or too little iodine in the diet are frequent causes. But not all patients with this disorder lose their hair, and the amount of hair loss doesn't match the severity of the disease. So other things may contribute to the problem: poor blood supply, too much cholesterol, incorrect processing of vitamin A, or local deposits of mucin--a substance that appears when the thyroid is under-producing. As in the case of other causes for hair loss, this condition requires careful evaluation.

We could go through several other diseases that can cause defects in or loss of your hair. For example, certain conditions lead to kinky or fine hair. Genetic disorders can make the hair shaft brittle because of low sulfur content. Some diseases affect the blood vessels, which in turn deliver too little blood to the scalp to give the hair proper nutrients. But technical discussions of many medical conditions are beyond our purpose in this book.

By discovering a cause for and treating temporary hair loss, doctors can often reverse radical changes in your appearance. Improving nutrition, changing grooming habits, or obtaining medication for infections and diseases are reasonable solutions for most of us. As you'll see in the next chapter, though, you'll need to seek different remedies if an evaluation points to permanent baldness.

3.
Permanent Hair Loss (Baldness)

The four most common causes of permanent hair loss other than disease are physical injury (cuts or burns), age, female-pattern hair loss, and male-pattern baldness. We'll spend more time on male-pattern baldness because it causes nearly 95 percent of all permanent, severe hair loss in men. Age alone or female-pattern hair loss usually causes only extensive diffuse thinning. Although they can create enough change in appearance to make some people seek a solution, neither is as severe as male-pattern baldness.

Physical Injury

If tissue in your scalp were damaged by cuts, deep radiation, or burns, your hair may not grow back. Destruction of hair follicles plus scar tissue combine to cause permanent loss. In this case, a hair addition or surgery is the only treatment. As we'll see in later chapters on surgery, scalp reductions (with or without tissue expansion) can remove the scarred, bald skin and "close up" areas of hair loss. We can also use Fleming/Mayer hair-flap surgery to place hair-bearing skin into areas from which we've removed damaged scalp.

Age

Your age affects how your hair grows. For example, at puberty some of your vellus hair becomes terminal hair. But with increasing age, you gradually lose scalp hair follicles--up to 20 percent between your 20th and 50th birthdays, and eight percent more over the next 30 years. Put another way, nearly 90 percent of men in their 20s have a full head of hair, but just over half retain it past the age of 40. Women also experience thinning of their scalp hair with age. But it typically occurs more slowly and diffusely (all over the scalp), rather than in noticeable patches as it does in men.

Hair loss from increasing age varies with the amount of testosterone present in the scalp, as well as with certain characteristics of your genetic makeup and immune system. Some heads thin slowly and steadily, whereas others may lose hair more rapidly and extensively. Overall, though, you have less chance of having a full head of hair as you get older.

Female-Pattern Hair Loss

This condition usually leads only to a general thinning of hair on the top and often on the sides of the scalp. Women rarely have bald spots on the crown and only occasionally have a receding front hairline. Typically, a woman will be in her 60s or 70s before reaching the full extent of her baldness, at which time her hair will also be finer and less luxuriant because of aging.

Because women do have male hormones, hormonal disorders can cause imbalances that lead to diffuse, but temporary, hair loss. Often, these changes result in other symptoms--acne will appear or get worse, hair may grow on the face and body, the sebaceous glands may become overactive and produce an oily scalp, and menstrual cycles may be irregular. Thus, if you're a woman with sudden, diffuse hair loss and other symptoms, you should see a doctor for evaluation. Once your hormone levels are back in balance, the hair loss will stop.

However, female-pattern hair loss is not a matter of temporary imbalances. Actual causes haven't been established, but because this loss is worse after menopause, male hormones and genetic signals probably play a role.

After menopause, women produce fewer female hormones but continue to produce male hormones, so the balance shifts toward the latter. Chemical interactions may take place in the hair follicles similar to those described below for male-pattern baldness.

Unfortunately, the most practical way a woman can deal with large, diffuse areas of baldness is to cover them with a hair addition. For female-pattern hair loss, neither injections nor applications of hormones and drugs to the scalp have proven very effective. Surgery is useful only if a woman has a male-pattern type of baldness-- with distinctly bald areas and plenty of donor hair on the sides of her head.

Male-Pattern Baldness

If you're genetically programmed for baldness, the follicles in your scalp will stop producing hair at a certain time in your life. They will continue their cycles of growth and rest, but growth is becoming shorter and resting longer. Also, each new hair produced is a little thinner and finer than the previous one. After a number of years, the follicles in your balding skin can produce only fine, vellus "fuzz"--easily visible under a microscope but nearly invisible to the naked eye. Your follicles remain intact but incapable of growing a normal head of hair.

Considerable research has established that male-pattern baldness (MPB) depends on three interrelated things: age, male hormones (androgens), and heredity. We've already pointed out how all balding tends to increase with age. The special pattern for MPB is familiar. It usually begins at the front of the head with a receding hairline. As it continues across the top of the scalp, a bald spot normally appears on the crown. Often, these areas meet to produce the final stage of MPB: a horseshoe-shaped rim of hair around the edge of the scalp.

The male hormone, testosterone, also plays a role in male-pattern hair loss. Males castrated before puberty-- and therefore no longer producing male hormones--

Male-Pattern Baldness Classifications

Class I: Front baldness only, with
or without a forward tuft.

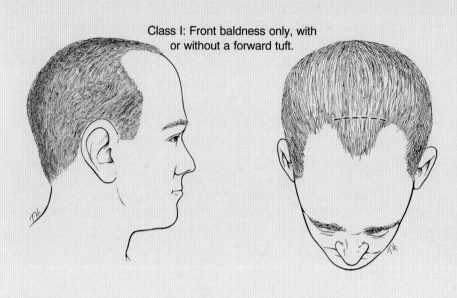

Class II: Front and midscalp baldness,
with no thinning of the crown.

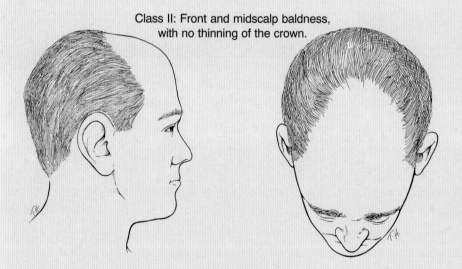

We classify balding patterns into four types. This classification helps us determine a person's ultimate pattern of baldness, so we can design treatment or surgery based on the final extent of your hair loss. Most balding men will eventually have Class III baldness. Thus, if you're young and have Class I baldness, we must carefully determine whether you'll stay as you are or progress to the Class II or III pattern. Early thinning of the midscalp or crown is an indicator.

Class III: Front to crown baldness

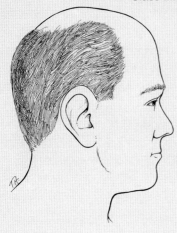
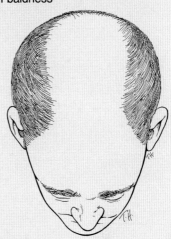

Class IV: Crown baldness only

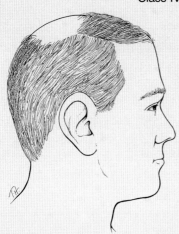
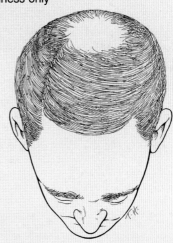

If we can't tell for sure how your baldness will progress, we typically recommend waiting until the pattern is more established. With time, the area between bald scalp and the hair that will never fall out becomes more distinct. We want to be certain that your final balding pattern is defined, so we don't use a donor area that continues balding after surgery. This pattern will also determine the ratio of good donor hair vs. the amount of baldness.

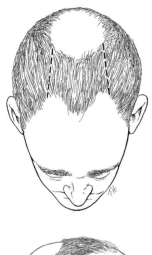

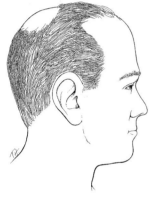

Fig. 3-1. Frontal and crown baldness. This pattern usually progresses to Class III and should be considered as such in evaluating patients for hair replacement surgery.

never experience male-pattern baldness. But even though testosterone clearly influences male-pattern baldness, no-one has found a difference between levels of testosterone within balding and non-balding men. The idea that bald men are particularly virile because they have more testosterone therefore isn't true.

In fact, male hormones alone don't make you bald. You must also be genetically predisposed to baldness. We've learned that balding starts when a genetic signal tells some of your follicles to convert testosterone to dihydrotestosterone, or DHT, through the action of the enzyme 5-alpha reductase. When enough DHT forms, these follicles slow down and stop producing terminal (normal) hairs. Apparently, certain follicles have receptors that are sensitive to DHT, so blocking the receptors may eventually be a way to cure pattern baldness.

This tendency to baldness appears to be hereditary, based on casual observation of bald men in particular families. Often (but not always), men have male-pattern baldness very similar to that of their fathers--or of their paternal or maternal relatives. But we still don't know for sure whether baldness comes from genes carried by men or by women. We believe that several genes must interact in the presence of male hormones to produce hair loss.

Once we understand the causes of baldness, we can discard some of the myths that people have created to explain it. For example, wearing tight hats, using mousse in our hair, or shampooing too frequently have nothing to do with permanent hair loss. Although these practices may temporarily damage hair, they don't alter the genetic progress in our hair cells. Instead of chasing obscure causes for hair loss, balding men are better served by learning how to cope with that loss. In the next chapter, we begin this process by discussing how to style your thinning hair for best appearance.

4.
Styling for Best Appearance

Sometimes, a change of hair style or slight improvement in your present style will distribute your hair more effectively over your thinning or bald areas. Obviously, styling can't give you back what you no longer have, but it can give you the appearance of having more hair— and thereby improve your self-image if you're bothered by baldness. Of course, blending or covering these areas to look natural can take considerable skill, depending on what you have to work with. That's why we recommend professional styling for all people who have problems with thinning hair. But if you have enough hair to comb at all, your stylist may be able to improve your appearance by using styling techniques to cover your thinning hair, receding hairline, or bald crown.

Combing and Brushing

A simple change in your combing technique may give your thinning hair more body and create the illusion of greater thickness. Using a soft-bristled brush, you can brush your hair gently forward from the nape of your neck to your forehead. We emphasize gentleness because vigorous backcombing may break or otherwise damage your hair, especially if it's thin in texture. After about a dozen strokes, reverse the direction of brushing-from your forehead back across your crown--and continue for another dozen strokes. Then, using the wide teeth of your comb to avoid snagging, style your hair in the usual way.

Some stylists recommend a "less is more" technique: staying away from combs, brushes, or parts and simply using the spread fingers on your hand to tousle your hair. The fingers give your hair just enough direction and more lift, which makes it look fuller. Another way of styling without a part is simply to shake your hair after showering and then lift it with your fingers, but otherwise leave it looking a bit "wild." This style can camouflage a receding hairline.

Shampooing and Conditioning

Whatever your hairstyle, frequent shampooing and conditioning are important to the health and appearance of your hair. How often you shampoo depends largely on when your hair becomes dirty from natural oils, buildup of hair products, or external pollutants and dust. Today's environment probably demands daily shampooing for most of us.

For best results, you should wash your hair carefully with a good pH shampoo. By good, we mean a mildly acidic pH of 4.5 to 5.1, which matches that of natural oils found on the scalp. Brushing your hair beforehand can effectively activate oil glands and loosen dead scales. Also, light massage may increase blood circulation, which can improve the flow of nutrients to your hair follicles. But opinions vary about the value of massage, and some dermatologists recommend against it because of its potential for damaging thin hair. Again, moderation is the key to proper technique.

Once you've wet your hair thoroughly with warm water, you can rub in the shampoo with your fingers. Don't scrape your skin with your fingernails; it doesn't need this irritation. Rinse well to avoid leaving residue on your scalp. Many stylists recommend a last rinse with cool water, which temporarily stops oil production in the sebaceous glands while helping to give your hair a shine.

Another necessary part of good hair care is conditioning. After shampooing, you should apply a high-quality, pH-balanced hair conditioner. (Most good conditioners today are balanced.) Sometimes, stylists recommend a slightly acidic cream conditioner for men with thinning hair because it causes the cuticle to "pucker" or expand, thus giving the hair more body. In any case, you should try to leave the conditioner on your hair for five minutes or so if possible and then rinse thoroughly with warm water. Rinsing is important. Because conditioners are oils, poor rinsing will leave your hair looking flat and oily. If you're in a hurry, don't skip the conditioning step. Even putting it on and taking it off is better than nothing.

Conditioners typically do one or more of four things to improve the surface layers of your hair--where most damage occurs. They flatten the hair cuticle (the outer layer of "shingles" covering the hair shaft) to increase sheen. They may decrease "fly-away" or dryness and often have agents that set your hair in place. Finally, they may contain "body builders" that improve sheen, repair surface cracks, or even move into the hair shaft to increase body. All of these improvements are especially helpful if your hair is thinning.

Conditioners work because their active ingredients carry a positive electrical charge which is attracted by the negative charge on newly shampooed hair. Thus, the conditioner can seep in under the cuticle layers and fill in any cracks or tears caused by chemicals or rough treatment. In addition, many conditioners contain protein additives that bond with the protein in your hair and mend snags, tears, or splits.

If your hair is particularly dry or oily, conditioners restore a natural balance to your follicles and promote healthy growth. But even "normal" hair needs conditioning because of the pollutants and other chemicals in our environment today. If you blow dry, bleach, dye, straighten, vigorously backcomb (tease), or expose your hair to a lot of sunlight, it will need more conditioning.

Moderate use of grooming aids may also improve your hair's appearance without damaging it. For example, gels and mousse increase volume, texture, and control without leaving your hair stiff or sticky. Mousse foams use negatively charged ingredients, which cause your negatively charged hair to fluff up and become fuller. At the same time, positively charged styling ingredients smooth your hair and make it shinier. In some cases, though, hair sprays and other dressings leave deposits on your hair which make it look dull. Oily groomers may also flatten your hair and emphasize thinning. If so, you may need to shampoo more often or use a stronger shampoo to remove these deposits.

You should also be very careful about coloring, curling, or straightening your hair at home. Alkaline-reducing agents used for curling or straightening, as well as hydrogen peroxide bleaches, can make your hair brittle and easy to break off. Stay away from solutions based on potassium hydroxide or aluminum hydroxide in particular. They cause your hair to "frizz," split, and tear. In the same way, using a hot comb or hot-oil treatments can loosen your hair from its follicles. The hot oil may even destroy follicles when it flows into them.

The key to proper hair care is moderation. Just because something is good for your hair doesn't mean using more of it is better. Shampooing, conditioning, and gently applying gels or sprays are all most of us need to keep our hair looking good and growing well.

Styles for Best Coverage

The shape of your face and head is particularly important to a flattering hair style. A professional stylist can analyze the bones of your cranium and face to help you understand why your hair may look better in one style or another.

Certain styles can mask or draw attention away from prominent features, such as a face that is too round, elongated, square, or triangular. In fact, the way you style your hair can help turn your facial shape into more of an oval, but with a broader curve at the top of your head. This shape is considered by many stylists to be ideal because it is suitable for nearly any style.

If you have a round face, for example, you'd want to avoid a style that frames your face, which would make it look even rounder and fuller. Instead, you could shape your hair with more height on top or make it slightly asymmetrical. These effects actually create the illusion of a more oval face.

A flat or slicked-down style will unfavorably accentuate a square or long face. If your face has one of these shapes, certain haircuts can add fullness to the sides of your head above your ears. In this case, your lower jaw seems narrower by comparison and, again, creates an oval effect.

If your face is triangular, you would want to avoid a style that sweeps the hair off your face and exaggerates the top or bottom "point." A style that works around your face by framing the area near your cheekbones can greatly reduce the sharpness of this facial shape.

Many stylists work "spherically" from a side view to fill in bare areas or to reduce the overall weight of your hair. Spot perming thin hair to give it more body can give you the overall shape you need for best results. Because males typically look better with a squarer, more blocked line, stylists will try to build height around the top of your head while keeping the sides relatively short. For this same reason, they also block the hair into a squarer pattern on the back of your neck rather than cutting in from the sides. These techniques give you the appearance of strength that is natural to men's styles.

Features of Your Face and Body

Most of us want to downplay any facial features that keep us from looking as good as possible. Hair styling can do just that. For example, a fringe of hair with varying lengths can soften a feature like wrinkled eyelids, which would look harder and more exaggerated next to a straight, blunt fringe. A side part can reduce the appar-

Fig. 4-1a and 4-1b. Coloring your hair can dramatically improve the appearance of thinning and/or graying hair.

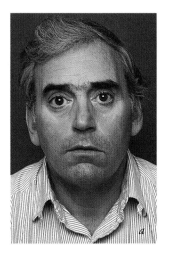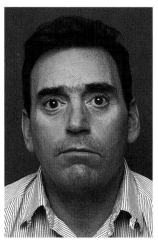

ent size of a nose that is large in proportion to other features of the face. Here, a center part would draw an observer's eye directly to the nose and accentuate its size. Stylists know many similar "tricks of the trade" to improve your appearance with hair cuts and arrangements.

Features of your body are important to hair styling, as well. If you have a small frame and body, a style with too much volume could make you look as though you're "all head." At the same time, a person who is large or obese would draw attention to his or her size with an overly full style.

Thinning Hair

For hair that has thinned out overall--usually without bald spots--stylists recommend a corrective hairstyle and haircut, plus techniques which add body to thin, fine hair. Most also suggest perming and, possibly, coloring for extra body and a younger appearance. The key to coloring is that darker is not better. Many men want dark colors because they consider them more youthful, but the contrast between hair and skin actually accentuates thinning spots. Instead, you should have semi-permanent colors that stay within the range appropriate to your skin tones, possibly with a bit of lighter highlighting on top. Special shampoos, conditioners, setting sprays, and hair thickeners can also increase sheen and the appearance of fullness, which is what you're striving for if you have thinning hair.

Lowering your part line a bit to take up more of your thick hair and bring it across the thinning area on top is a good way to start. Of course, you don't want to go too far below the normal part line--usually calculated to extend upward from the junction of the middle and outer thirds of your eyebrow. An abnormally low part will make you look unnatural. Also, you must wait up to ten months until this "re-parted" hair grows long enough for full coverage (five to six inches).

Your hair stylist can then determine what sort of cut will appear thicker on top. Typically, you'll want less bulk on the sides, so your thicker hair will blend more with the fine hair on top and give you a "balanced" look. We recommend a "layered" cut, whereby groups of hair are cut in equal lengths but adjacent groups have varying length. Careful layering only on top will help camouflage exposed areas of scalp and give your hair more body.

Once your cut is complete, most stylists apply a good setting spray to hold your hair in place without making it stiff or sticky. Then, they add a hair-thickener product, blow-dry your hair to give it "lift"--especially at the partline and front hairline, and use hair spray to add final body and holding power.

Obviously, with extensive thinning, you can't expect styling to cover your entire scalp. But you can keep your remaining hair healthy by shampooing regularly to remove oils and buildup of styling products. You can use the techniques and materials described above to give your hair a thicker appearance. And, when combing your hair, you can employ the fine teeth on the comb to keep the shafts closer together for better coverage. With extensive baldness, you're much better off having a nice haircut around your remaining hair rather than trying to comb a few lonely strands across the top. Although these methods won't restore hair, they certainly will give you a better appearance.

Receding Hairline

Most men over the age of 21 have receding hairlines, so your recessions are normal. Yet, there's no need to emphasize a receding hairline unless you want to. For example, if you normally comb your hair straight back without a part, you can do one of three things to make your recessions less prominent. First, you can part your hair in the middle and sweep it to either side in order to cover the bald areas. Or you might try styling your front hairline more forward. This method, usually referred to as a "Caesar" style, requires some care to avoid the appearance of bangs. You should especially avoid slicking

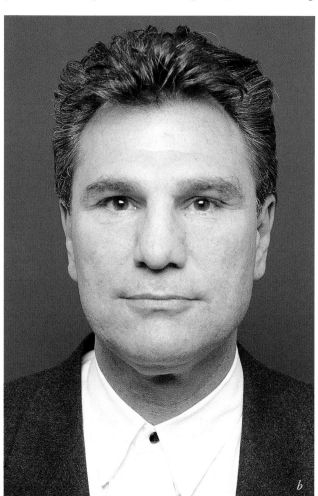

Fig. 4-2a and 4-2b. Proper styling helps draw attention away from a receding hairline.

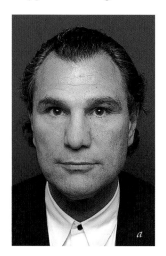

down your hair and combing it flat against your scalp. Most stylists recommend instead creating lift in the front line of hair with a mild permanent wave, then moving the hair slightly forward to create the illusion of fullness. Finally, if you have long, straight hair, you can change to a side part and comb your hair across the recessions.

If your hair has receded farther on one side than the other, you can part your hair on the side with the least recession. The best approach is to make the part high enough to conceal the bald area on the parted side and then comb your hair over the other bald section. If both recessions are the same, you'll want your part to be on the side where your hair looks best.

Thinning or Bald Crown

Unfortunately, the hair in front of a balding crown grows forward and therefore tends to expose rather than hide it. Attempts to comb your existing hair over the crown usually fail, because this natural pull makes it droop toward your forehead. Thus, to conceal a thinning crown, you must let the hair in front and on the sides grow long enough to comb it over your bald or thinning area.

Once your hair grows to the proper length, you have two options for styling: no part and side part. With no part, you simply begin at the front of your head and comb the hair straight back to the nape of your neck. The hair from the top and sides will meet in a kind of "V" at the back of your head.

As with generally thinning hair, a side part may need to be a bit lower if you want to comb your hair over a bald crown. Otherwise, the technique is straightforward, except that any hair parted and combed across the head tends to want to lie straight across, or slightly forward along the contour of the scalp.

To redirect your hair across the bald area, a professional stylist will probably begin by drying and brushing it into position. The stylist knows that when you pull up on your brush with a section of wet hair and blow hot air in front of the brush and onto the hair roots, your hair reacts by creasing toward the direction in which you're brushing. He also knows not to overdry your hair because overdrying causes the hair to become "tired" and shapeless. A good rule of thumb is that if your hair looks dry but feels cool to the touch, you're done. While adding height to both sides of the part and frontal outline, this technique allows you to comb your hair over the crown.

Of course, as soon as your hair gets wet--from perspiration, rain, or shampooing--the crease relaxes and has to be redone. So, to get "permanent" redirection of your hair, a stylist has to use permanent waving. In this case, perm rods rolled toward the crown substitute for the styling brush. By using large rods, the stylist gets direction and body but not curly hair. You can then comb your newly permed hair over your crown, because it will grow according to the direction in which it was rolled.

Front-to-Crown Baldness

With Class III baldness, your hair has receded to the point where all you have left is a strip of growth beginning above your ears and continuing around to the back of your head. The top, for the most part, is bald. If you have heavy, abundant hair on your part side, however, you may be able to grow it long enough to provide some coverage of your scalp. Of course, you must recognize that this styling won't work if you subject it to much wind or any water. In other words, it has to be maintained and renewed if it is to keep anything like a natural look.

This hair styling technique is more effective if you still have a fuzzy growth on your frontal scalp because your professional stylist can use it as a cushion for hair taken from the side and combed across. A cushion raises your recombed hair and gives it a more natural look. Of course, as for thinning hair (see above), you also must be careful not to place your part unnaturally low while trying to "shift" hair to the top of your head.

The first step in restyling your hair is to allow the remaining hair to grow all one length. When it has grown long enough, your stylist can lower your natural part up to an inch below where it was and begin "training" this 1-inch-wide strip of hair to extend across your bald scalp. Again, because your hair grows only one-half to one inch per month, it will take up to 10 months to get the five or six inches of length you need for coverage.

This area of improvised hair isn't enough to make your hair on top as thick as the hair growing at the sides and back. As a result, your stylist will still need to cut your hair effectively and use various hair products to make it thicker and fuller. As we mentioned earlier, most stylists recommend against extra-long or bulky hair at the sides and back of your head; it actually emphasizes thinness on top and may even give you a "clown-like" appearance. Also, using length to try to make up for thinness will usually work against you because longer hair tends to flatten and become limp under its own weight, thus actually giving you less body.

After cutting your hair properly, your stylist will probably set it and add a hair thickener to give it more body. Blow drying to get height on both sides of your part and a good hair spray will finish off your new look. Some stylists frown on hair sprays, but moderate use helps to bond your hair, hold the style, and add body of its own. With the right techniques, even starting from a fully bald condition, hair styling can often give you enough coverage to conceal some of your baldness and to improve your appearance.

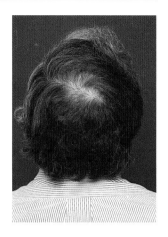

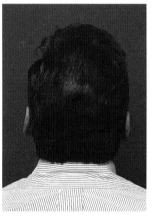

Fig. 4-3a (top) and 4-3b (above). This gentleman, the same man in 4-1a and 4-1b, camouflages his balding crown with coloring and proper hair styling.

Permanent Waving

A waving solution penetrates the cortex layer of your hair and "breaks down" its normal straight growth so it can take on a curl. Large perm rods create softer (larger) curls or waves, and smaller rods produce tighter, smaller curls.

In most cases, your stylist will want to use a permanent to put body and lift into both sides of your part, as well as to lift up the front of your hair for better coverage. Using large perm rods allows body and lift without causing the hair to "shrivel" and reveal more bald area on top. One approach is to keep the wave uniform on top and sides by using large setting rods all over, or at least the largest possible rods depending on the amount of hair available.

Once your hair is rewetted and rolled, your stylist will apply a permanent-wave solution to all parts of the rolled hair. The solution will vary in strength depending on whether your hair is damaged (mild), normal, or resistant (strong). After a certain amount of time, which varies with the type of solution, a curled pattern will appear. As mentioned above, this pattern occurs when your hair breaks down enough to take the shape of the rod it is on.

You'll then get a thorough rinse with warm water and a neutralizing solution on the perm rods in all areas of your hair. After five minutes, your stylist will remove the rods and gently rub the remaining solution through your hair. A few minutes later, the neutralizer is thoroughly washed out of your hair with warm water and finished with a few seconds of cooler water. Your hair is now ready for styling.

If you're resistant to the idea of permanent waving, it's probably because you've seen a "bad job." Although tightly curled or kinky hair does give the appearance of better coverage, especially with hair transplants (see Chapter 9), it may not be right for the contours of your face and head. Thus, we don't necessarily recommend these tighter styles.

It's also important to work with stylists who are sensitive to the potential dangers of permanent waving. For example, your hair has to be in condition for permanent waving; if it is discolored or broken, you shouldn't have a permanent until proper conditioning restores it to healthy growth. To avoid damage, a stylist must handle your "permed" hair gently, use the right tension when winding your hair on rollers, and apply solution of the right strength for your hair's condition. Finally, he must rinse chemicals thoroughly from your hair so no odors remain and the curl doesn't relax. Otherwise, you may actually lose hair from permanent waving or, at least, be dissatisfied with its results.

Some men are uncomfortable with the idea of getting a permanent for their hair. If you feel this way, you may find comfort in knowing that men from all walks of life regularly visit their hair salons for a "perm." A permanent can create a natural, wavy look while redirecting your hair over sparse areas of your scalp. If your hair is thinning unevenly, stylists can "spot perm" the thinning areas to create the illusion of more bulk in smaller sections rather than trying to create an overall permed style. The effectiveness and flexibility of permanent waving highly recommend it as part of your styling routine.

Styles and Methods to Avoid

One basic piece of advice we can give you is to avoid combing your hair in a direction opposite from the one in which it lies naturally. Thus, if your partline or other sections of your hair will lie only in one direction, modify your hairstyle to correspond with the way the hair is growing. Otherwise, it may be hard to manage and look unnatural.

In addition, certain styles seem to call attention to a balding condition rather than masking it. As we've suggested, lowering your part too close to one ear is a classic instance. So is parting your hair at the nape of your neck and sweeping it forward. Professionally lowered parts, such as those in the styles recommended above, won't upset the symmetry of your head and face.

We've mentioned the negative effects of exceptionally long or bulky side hair. A variation--allowing your sideburns to grow down to your jawline--will also emphasize your baldness. In other words, it's usually better to live with baldness, or to seek another method of covering or replacing it, than to adopt "desperate measures."

Apart from particular styles, you should avoid some methods of hair care which damage thinning hair. Obvious cases are overbleaching, over-dyeing, over-straightening, and over-perming. These techniques dry and break hair, so they are especially harmful if your hair is already stressed by thinning. Razor cutting can also damage your hair by tearing apart your hair cuticles, which causes dullness and tangling as well as a tendency to lie flat (without body). If your technician uses a razor to cut your hair, he or she must have proper training, possibly including certification by one of the schools that teach this technique. The razor should be used especially sparingly on bleached or permed hair.

You also need to use brushes, combs, and hair dryers with care. For example, stiff nylon brushes and fine-toothed combs can damage kinky or wet hair because they tend to "yank apart" curls or tangles. Excessive backcombing with fine teeth can actually strip off the cuticles from your hair shafts and therefore cause premature breaking and split ends. Hair dryers can burn or break your hair if you hold them too close to the hair's surface--less than six inches away. Again, gentle use of the normal "tools" for hair styling will give you the best results.

If you are balding, the best approach is to choose a professional stylist and depend on him or her to get the results you want. Styling your own hair rarely works well in areas of severe thinning or balding. Your goal is to obtain the best possible appearance within the limits established by the thinness of your hair. If you require a fuller head of hair, you must look into hair additions or surgical solutions for hair replacement.

5.
Non-surgical Hair Additions

Hair additions have come a long way in the past 20 years. The traditional toupee had a foundation made of natural fiber that would shrink and break down under normal wearing conditions. Now, we have highly sophisticated, manufactured materials that repel perspiration and oils and can hold up under modern attachment methods. Cottons and silk gauze have given way to polyesters and nylon, combined with silicones and polymers that make parts and foundations look like natural skin. As a result, high-quality hair additions are a safe, reasonable treatment for balding men who are unable or unwilling to seek a permanent solution through surgery.

Choosing Synthetic or Human Hair

In the past, you'd have had very little choice here, because synthetic "hair" was a poor substitute for the real thing. Human hair had markedly better texture, color, range of styles, and resistance to heat. It allowed the wearer to change styles himself and to participate in activities that subjected the hair addition to heat, such as hot showers, saunas, and hot tubs. Today, perhaps because of its past superiority, many hair replacement centers continue to recommend human hair except for shades of gray and white. Gray or white human hair yellows over time, so synthetic fibers are necessary to keep a natural look.

When synthetics were first introduced in the late 60s and early 70s, they had a high-gloss sheen which wouldn't match human hair. Their coarse texture, obvious color, and reflectivity made them useless for all but the cheapest of hair additions. They were also nearly impossible to style and wouldn't hold their shape. But now they look so much more natural that it's difficult even for the experts to differentiate them from human hair. That's one reason the new synthetic fibers make up well over half of all hair additions purchased in the United States.

Still, as you can see in the comparative panel, there are differences between synthetic fibers and human hair. Your choice depends on your lifestyle and personal demands. It's wise to consult with a specialist who carries both types, so you can get an unbiased opinion. Then, select the type of hair which suits you best. Or, as some

SYNTHETIC HAIR VS. HUMAN HAIR

SYNTHETIC HAIR	HUMAN HAIR
• Durable; outlasts human hair.	• Wears out, breaks, splits.
• Duller, less bouncy, less soft and natural.	• More natural, elastic, springy, and reflective.
• Retains style up to 3 months; easy to shape after washing or swimming.	• Requires extensive styling after washing or swimming.
• Doesn't fade from sun or chlorination; doesn't need dyeing.	• Oxidizes in 3-12 months; requires dyeing to maintain color.
• "Frizzes" under high heat; newest synthetics can withstand hot tubs.	• Resists extreme temperatures; will burn if exposed directly to flame.
• Not as absorbent as human hair; shampoos and conditioners for human hair are not compatible.	• Absorbs moisture from sink, shower, or pool; allows use of standard shampoos and conditioners for daily care.
• Dries faster; less matting or tangling.	• Dries slowly; may tangle.
• Can be hand-washed in a sink but requires special cleaning solution.	• Best washed with solvents by a professional.
• Best for gray or white hair, but other colors less natural than human hair.	• More natural-looking colors other than gray or white.

people do, you might keep both types, using the more durable synthetic hair for swimming, sports, or other outdoor recreation and human hair for day-to-day activities.

Some salons have tried to capture the "best of both worlds" by mixing human and synthetic hair in the same addition, but you may not be satisfied with the results after a few months. At that point, the salon will usually have to dye the natural hair to reverse discoloration from sun and water. Unfortunately, the synthetic fiber won't take the dye, so you're likely to be left with a multi-colored, unnatural-looking hair addition.

Types of Hair Additions

Hair additions are available in two basic types: ready made (stock) or custom made.

Ready-Made — The average ready-made hair addition costs between $450 and $750. It is intended to fit the most popular colors, sizes, and styles of an average client. For example, most males wear a left part, so finding a right part in a ready made is almost impossible. Ready-mades also come in limited colors. If you have dark hair, such as a plain, off-black color, you can find a match much easier than blondes and redheads can. Ready-mades especially lack highlighting—a number of lighter shades of color that most men have in their growing hair.

Ready-made hair additions are deficient in another crucial area: the natural look that comes with proper fit and personalized styling. With literally thousands of shapes and contours of the balding area, it's unlikely that you will get the same fit as in a custom-made addition. Also, a ready made usually has too much hair, and technicians can do only so much to personalize its style to an individual wearer. It often looks artificial, especially if you're older. The hairline may be too low or too full, even after cutting. Special shapes, such as a naturally receding hairline, are difficult to get. And a slightly thinning look — also natural to men of 40 or older — probably won't be possible with a ready-made. A technician's typical improvements, such as adding some gray or slightly changing the design, usually aren't enough to fully satisfy a wearer.

Custom-Made — The best quality hair additions are custom made—matched precisely with your hair color, shaped to fit your head, and styled to match the contours of your face. Hair replacement centers or full-service hair salons offer this service. A technician takes a mold or casting of your head in order to craft a foundation that fits its contours and mark off a proposed hairline. The technician then hand-ties individual human, synthetic, or blended hairs to the foundation. Proper hair thickness, curl, direction, length, knotting techniques, and careful matching of colors and highlighting with samples of your hair all ensure a more natural-looking hair style than in the ready-made addition.

Your initial cost for a custom hair addition will be $1,200 to $3,000, depending on the materials, overhead in your geographical area, and experience of the specialist who constructs it. In most cases, you should allow six to twelve weeks from the date of your order for delivery, plus time for styling and final adjustments. A replacement addition, which doesn't require a mold or any of the initial consultations, should run about $800 to $2,000. If the foundation is in good repair, some centers will replace only the hair for $200 to $500. This less expensive alternative might give your addition six months to a year of extra life.

Selecting a Hair Addition Foundation

A hair addition foundation is important because it holds the replacement hair in position and is the part of the addition that fits next to your head. Thus, it needs to be comfortable, light, strong, and able to allow scalp perspiration to evaporate, so your head remains relatively cool.

Today, foundations come in four basic types: molded plastic or fiberglass, polyurethane or silicone (resembling skin), fiber-based mesh, and combinations of mesh and skin-like materials. Molded plastic and fiberglass foundations either have air holes for ventilation or are solid. They vary from thick, rigid materials to soft, bendable epoxy. They're designed for daily wear but are removed during the evening. If the foundation has ventilation holes, you would attach it with double-sided tape. If it is solid, you would press it firmly down on your head so the vacuum created underneath would hold it on. This suction attachment requires a perfect fit, so solid foundations should be custom made. At one time, molded plastic or fiberglass was the most popular type of foundation. Now it has fallen out of favor because it is heavy, hot, and limited to certain styles. Its wearer also can't use a more permanent method of attachment because cleaning the scalp underneath it is almost impossible.

The polyurethane or silicone foundation looks like a "scalp," with texture and color very close to that of your own skin. Manufacturers fuse individual synthetic hairs into this foundation to create styles which can be ready made or custom made. If you live in a cooler climate and don't have a particularly active lifestyle, you may like this kind of foundation because it appears as though the entire scalp is your own. Polyurethane and silicone offer especially good results if you don't want much hair in the addition. Although these foundations are much lighter and thinner than those of molded plastic or fiberglass, they are still poorly ventilated and are therefore hot to wear.

Fiber-based mesh foundations are the most popular today because they offer more comfort and easier access to the scalp for cleaning if they are attached more permanently. Nylon (monofilament) and polyester are commonly used materials. They can be combined with silicone or polyurethane sections to give the appearance of skin at the hairline, crown, or part. Mesh foundations also lend themselves to "hand-tied" or "stranded" hair. This technique allows individual hairs to be pulled

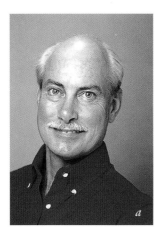
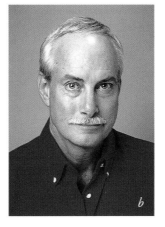
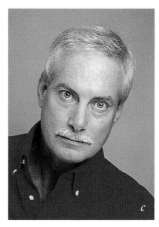

Figs. 5-1a through 5-1d. Gentleman phasing into larger hair additions for a natural, gradual effect.
5-1e. Different style in hair addition.

through the mesh and then tied, glued, or crimped to hold them in place. Because each hair moves freely at the foundation, the addition looks natural and is easily styled or restyled. It allows special blending of gray or other colors, as well as varying length or thickness on certain areas of your scalp. Mesh foundations are available in ready made and custom made additions, using human hair, synthetics, or blends.

Prices of hair additions vary not only with the choice of foundation materials but also with the type of knotting, which the industry calls ventilation technique. People often believe that the addition with the most hair will be the most expensive, but in reality the opposite is true. The less hair put into each knot tied to the foundation, the more expensive the addition. Using one hair at a time in knotting results in the most natural look, so this "single-hair ventilation" is the most expensive process in the industry. Because various knotting techniques are available, you should allow your specialist to choose the one most appropriate for your addition.

Crafting the Hairline

Carefully crafted hairlines continue to be crucial in order to achieve a natural look with a hair addition. In most cases, balding men have little or no hair to blend with the addition along the hairline, so specialists have to use other techniques to achieve this natural appear-

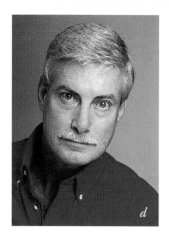
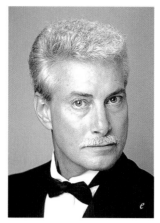

ance. The oldest method came from Max Factor in Hollywood: placing a fine lace material at the front section of a hair addition. By matching this lace to the skin tone and applying it to the scalp with liquid adhesive, the specialist could make it look like hair was coming directly out of the scalp.

These lace fronts worked fine for Hollywood's short-term use in individual movies, but they broke down easily under daily wear by the average man on the street. Consequently, they nearly disappeared from public use until fine nylon monofilament and polyester blends surfaced during the last few years. They're now becoming popular again, but they still wear more quickly than other foundation materials and are not yet suited for more permanently attached hair additions.

Fortunately, hair specialists today have other ways to refine the hairline.

Color — Coloring or highlighting the front edge of the hairline matches it closer to the wearer's skin color, camouflaging the contrast between skin and hair.

Short hairs — Designers can cut the front edge of the hairline so very short hairs are directed forward. When tapered properly, these hairs remain flush to the hairline and conceal the edge of the foundation.

Short, curly hairs — Many nonbalding men have fine "baby" hairs at the hairline which are slightly curlier than their more dominant, straight terminal hairs. Placing a very fine front edge of these "baby" hairs on a hair addition softens its normally solid front line.

Thinning — Natural hair is thinner at the front edge of the hairline. Thinning an addition to reduce weight and density along its hairline creates a much softer, more natural look.

Curl or wave — For swept-back styles without a lace front, a stylist places a wave in the hair so it curves forward a bit from the foundation before starting back toward the crown. This technique creates more fullness or a slightly higher look at the front hairline and therefore offers better coverage.

Recessions — Designing recessions into the hair addition will give the hairline a much more natural appearance. The wearer's age and existing hair are keys to the proper amount of recession, but a conservative approach usually gives the best results (fig.5-1).

Choosing Proper Color and Texture

Proper hair color is one of the most important aspects of a natural-looking hair addition. As mentioned, a person's natural hair color is often a blend of up to eight different colors. At the back and sides you want the addition's hair color to be the same as your growing hair, but in most cases the top and front should be lighter. Even people with black hair require lighter colors in the front to soften the hairline and appearance. Highlighting provides this natural look.

Color charts or rings guide the choice of hair that is added to the top, front, or other areas of the ready-made hair addition. For custom mades, the specialist will take a sample of your own hair to get the proper match. If you have a graying pattern in your hair, the percentage of gray will vary in different areas. Thus, a specialist must carefully consider your pattern in creating a hair addition, usually ordering slightly more gray than you have to show the natural progress of your graying over the time that you will use the addition.

Regarding texture, if your own hair is very fine,

you'll be better off with slightly coarser, stronger hair in the addition. It won't feel too coarse as long as the specialist avoids too much thickness or density in the addition. Although the finest human hair is most expensive, it's not always better. Fine human hair is weaker and cannot always stand up to recolorings and perms. It breaks, sheds, and tangles easier than hair with a slightly coarser texture. We recommend consulting with a specialist about the best texture for your addition.

Once the hair addition itself is complete, your stylist must decide on a way to attach it to your head. Numerous methods of attaching hair additions have recently come into vogue, but they fall into two basic categories: to the skin and to existing hair. If your addition is properly made, any of the following attachment techniques is possible.

Attaching an Addition to Your Scalp

Attaching an addition directly to the skin works best only if you have no thinning hair growing on your bald scalp or if you're willing to shave this hair before fitting the addition. If thinning hair covers the skin, adhesives work less well, and removal of the addition can pull this hair out, causing further loss. Besides suction or vacuum fitting, mentioned earlier for molded plastic or fiberglass foundations, the most common ways to attach an addition to the skin are double-sided adhesive tape, surgical adhesive, surgical suturing, and tunnel grafts.

Double-Sided Tape — Clear double-sided tape is a very common way to secure standard hair additions. The tape comes in variably shaped strips, fitting easily to the rounded form of the hair addition base. You attach tape to the front, back, and sides of the base. Then, you position the hair addition correctly and gently press it onto the scalp. For hair additions with combed-back styles on lace-mesh foundations, you may use a spirit gum to secure the hairline. For less noticeable locations, some tape has velcro on one side. The wearer places the adhesive sides of the tape at matching positions on the hair addition base and the scalp, then "velcroes" the base onto his head. This system operates much like velcro fasteners on clothing.

Modern adhesive tapes are very effective as long as you have no hair or very little growing hair on your head. They're quick and easy to use but not the most secure method of attachment. You risk dislodgement if you sleep, shower, or swim in your hair addition. The tape must be replaced every two to three days — more frequently in humid climates or for oily scalps — and rotated to prevent sore spots on your scalp.

Surgical Adhesives — Some salons shave a narrow band around the top of your fringe hair to establish a base for a ring of surgical adhesive. They then apply adhesive, much like caulking, in a circle around the top of your head. All that remains is to position the hair addition and press it down onto the ring of adhesive, causing it to bond temporarily with the scalp.

Surgical adhesive is very secure but requires a visit to the salon every four to five weeks to have it removed and redone. That's about how long the adhesive holds its "sticking power," after which your hair addition will start to slip. You may experience more oil build-up and heat because the thick ring of adhesive can block air flow from the sides of the addition.

Hygiene can also be a problem. You must rely on shampooing and flushing water through the hair addition to remove oils and bacteria from your scalp. Impurities tend to build up along the back edge of the hair addition, causing an unpleasant odor. Of course, you get a thorough cleaning every four weeks or so when you go in to have the adhesive replaced.

Surgical Suturing — You may have heard surgical suturing called "implantation," but no hair is implanted as part of the procedure. Rather, a doctor sews a ring of sutures into the scalp, leaving a series of exposed loops above the surface of the skin (fig. 5-2, 5-3). The sutures, a Teflon-coated stainless steel like those used in heart

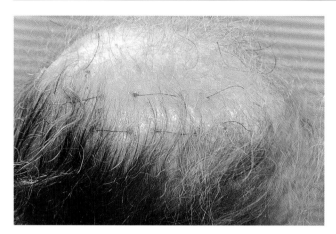

Fig. 5-2 (left). Suture method of continuous sutures placed all around the balding area.

Fig. 5-3 (below). Ring suture technique.

Fig. 5-4 (bottom). Spiral suture technique.

surgery, are chosen to reduce the possibility of infection. Once the sutures are in place, a salon technician can attach a hair addition simply by sewing it to them. Because the addition is anchored to the sutures, rather than to your growing hair, it doesn't require the inconvenience and cost of regular visits to the salon for tightening. On the other hand, it is very difficult to clean the scalp under the addition. Collected oil and bacteria often cause discomfort and an unpleasant odor.

A variation of this technique makes cleaning your scalp easier. The doctor starts with sutures at the top center of your head and spirals out toward the fringe of your naturally growing hair (fig. 5-4). In this case, the salon sews individual wefts of artificial hair to each loop, starting at the top center of your head and moving outward until they cover the bald area. They then blend the hair together in a natural style. This cleaner approach also lets more air reach the scalp and is therefore cooler. The disadvantage is your artificial hair will not be as dense as a full hair addition.

Once your hair addition is on, it becomes a part of you. You swim, shower, and sleep with it because you can't take it off. Your only requirement is an annual checkup, during which the salon can check the condition of your hair addition and replace hair if necessary. Synthetic hair is probably your best bet in this case; it's washable, durable, and capable of returning quickly to

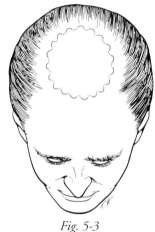

Fig. 5-3

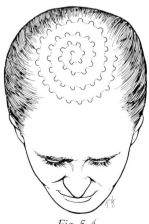

Fig. 5-4

its original style after wear. Because you wear the hair addition continuously, choosing the highest quality of replacement hair is especially important, if you want it to last.

Although the convenience and relative permanence of suturing sound good, significant disadvantages of both procedures have caused many doctors to recommend against them. We have found that more complaints are registered concerning suture-attached hair additions than any other form of hair-replacement technique. Often, people are uncomfortable while sleeping because of pressure on the surgical loops, as well as the possibility of the sutures "migrating" and throwing the hair addition off center. Also, an accident can tear the sutures through the scalp, causing damage that would have to be repaired and, possibly, some scarring. Most important is the frequent occurrence of infection where the sutures enter the scalp. Although the infection can be controlled by medication, it often spreads, causing serious and permanent damage. Treatment usually requires removal of the hair addition and sutures.

Costs for suturing are high. The surgical procedure itself will run you between $1,000 and $1,750. On top of that are the costs for the hair addition and its maintenance. Depending on where you live and the quality of service, your total might be as much as $3,000 to $4,000. Because of the high costs and risks involved, we don't recommend suturing as a method of attachment for hair additions.

Surgical "Tunnel Grafts" — A plastic surgeon can remove skin grafts from another part of your body, form them into small loops, and surgically attach them to the scalp skin in order to create tunnels—usually two at the front and one at the back. You can then easily and securely snap a hair addition equipped with clips at matching locations to the grafts. The hair addition stays on straight but can be removed with three quick snaps.

Surgeons commonly remove a strip of skin from behind your ear to form the loops. This technique is superior to suturing because it doesn't cause infection. The skin loop comes from your own body and is not rejected as a foreign substance. Of course, with skin loops sticking up from the top of your scalp, you would not want to take the hair addition off in public. Some doctors also worry that a strong tug or accident could rip the hair addition through the skin grafts, although the clips would probably give way first. In addition, swimming, showering, or sleeping with the hair addition attached could cause irritation or infection.

Most doctors recommend tunnel grafts only for people who want their scalp covered all the time, such as those with burns or scarring. Together with a durable hair addition made of high-quality synthetic hair, grafts allow almost continuous public wear, as long as you're careful about scalp hygiene. If you wanted to reverse the process at any time, scars would remain after a doctor snipped through the loops of skin to remove the grafts.

Because tunnel grafts require a surgical procedure by a skilled physician, you're likely to pay as much as $3,000 for complete service: consultations, surgery, and the hair addition. Although you wouldn't have to visit a salon for regular tightening or retying, your hair addition would probably need routine servicing, such as repairs, retinting, or styling. The usual cost for such visits is $25 to $50, depending on your location.

Attaching an Addition to Your Hair

Many salons and hair-replacement centers recommend attaching a hair addition directly to your naturally growing hair because they consider this method either more convenient or more secure. The most common types of this form of attachment are clips and barrettes, cabling or weaving, and fusion.

Clips or Barrettes — Clips or barrettes are permanently attached to the hair addition unit and then are secured to the growing hair on your head. For full frontal baldness, tape must replace clips along the front hairline. A common variety is the guillotine clip, so named

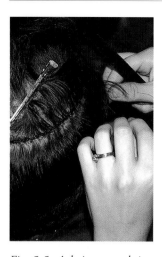

Fig. 5-5. A hair weave being performed. Hair addition is sewn to braid and must be retightened every four to six weeks.

because you place your own hair across its base and then bring down an "arm" that crimps the hair in place as it locks into the base. Others may have comb-like teeth that secure the hair addition to growing hair. While not as permanent as some methods of attachment, clips are quick and easy to attach and remove. As your hair grows, you can retighten them with little effort.

Cabling or Weaving — These two methods are virtually the same technique. Cabling requires weaving a thin nylon line into the hair addition base and into the growing hair next to bald areas. The two lines of woven thread are then knotted together with additional pieces of nylon "cable" at several locations around the head. To prepare for weaving, you grow your hair long on the sides, so the technician can braid it around the circumference of your bald area (fig. 5-5). He then sews nylon line through the base of your hair addition and into your braided hair.

Cabling or weaving is very secure and still allows you to clean the scalp underneath the hair addition. The gaps between points of attachment allow oils and bacteria to flush off the top of the scalp and also leave room for ventilation and cooling. Assuming the cable is tightly tied, you can sleep, swim, and exercise in your hair addition. Periodically, you must return to the salon for regular adjustments as your growing hair pulls the addition away from your scalp.

At salons which use cabling or weaving for attachment, the initial service will likely include both the hair addition and attachment. The total cost will range from $250 for some ready-made additions to more than $1,500 for a custom-made one. Periodic maintenance visits, including haircutting and styling, are likely to cost you $40 to $60 or more, depending on where you live.

Fusion — Fusion uses adhesive plus hooks and eyes to attach the hair addition. The hooks attach permanently at several points around your addition. Then, a stylist pulls your growing hair through the eye, twists it, and bonds it to itself. By looping one hook through each of the eyes, the stylist can quickly secure the addition to your head. You can take your hair addition off simply by opening the hooks and eyes. You can sleep, swim, shower, and exercise in your addition if you wish to, yet easily take it off for servicing, as well as to clean your scalp. Of course, because continuous wearing can reduce the life of the addition, most salons recommend you remove it at bedtime. Again, as with cabling or weaving, you must go in for servicing and rebonding about every five to six weeks. The interval depends on how quickly your natural hair continues to grow. A stylist will snip off the fused ends of your hair at these sessions and then reloop and rebond your growing hair to the rings. Costs for maintenance visits are comparable to those for weaving or cabling.

Getting a Natural-Looking Hair Addition

A natural look depends on the product itself, the hair-addition specialist, and you.

The Product — A good hair addition has a properly fitted, comfortable base and hair of the right density, texture, and color to blend with your growing hair. It attaches securely, and the hairline and style must complement your features. It gives you ready access for proper hygiene, such as daily shampooing and rinsing. Above all, it matches your lifestyle and activities.

The Specialist — The very best product available isn't wearable without the proper design and planning for your individual needs. Once you've chosen a salon or replacement center, carefully plan the "look" you want to achieve, so no surprises await you (fig. 5-6, 5-7). Ask to meet other people who have bought hair additions from the specialist to ensure he or she can give you the results you expect. Make sure you communicate clearly with the specialist about cutting, styling, and maintenance after the purchase. Together, these precautions will assure you of high-quality service and a natural appearance.

You — If you're not dedicated to caring properly

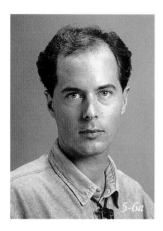

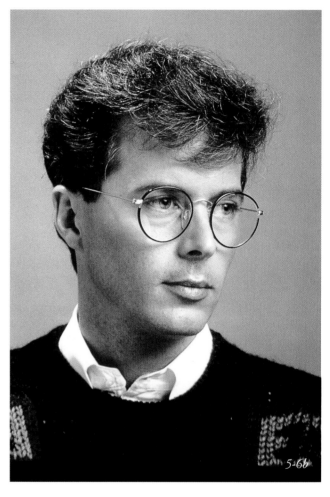

Fig. 5-6a (above), 5-6b (right), 5-7a (opposite left), 5-7b (opposite right). High quality hair additions are a good alternative for men who are unwilling to seek a permanent solution to their baldness through surgery.

for your hair addition, even the most expensive model will quickly begin to look unnatural. Sometimes, the foundation needs repair. Because your natural hair continues to grow, cabled, woven, or fused hair additions need tightening at regular intervals — usually every five to six weeks. Of course, you also need haircuts and styling to keep your growing hair blended with the replacement hair.

You also must stress good scalp hygiene if you want to be satisfied with a hair addition. Most centers recommend washing the scalp by lifting up the front of the addition and applying an astringent to break down bacteria and oil buildup. Some suggest a biodegradable

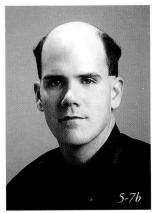

5-7b

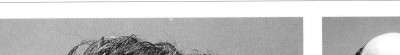

5-7a

soap, which easily combines with plain water. If your addition is properly vented, rinsing will naturally flush all impurities away from your scalp. Together with regular shampooing and rinsing of your hair, these techniques will ward off discomfort and unpleasant odors.

Other Forms of Hair Additions

Hair Integration or Intensification — Hair integration works only when there's enough naturally growing hair — usually close to three-quarters of the original growth — to anchor replacement wefts (strips) placed into sections of thinning hair. The process uses a base of silk webbing with holes about one-quarter inch in diam-

COMMON ERRORS IN USING HAIR ADDITIONS

- Buying an addition that is too dark for your skin tones or that has an improper hairstyle for your features, existing hair, age, or lifestyle.

- Wearing hair that is too thick or too long.

- Flattening the addition too much and wearing the hair too straight.

- Attaching the removable addition too hurriedly, so it rests unnaturally on your head or shifts with wear.

- Pulling a more permanently attached addition down lower on your forehead to tighten it after several weeks of wear. This gives you a top-heavy look.

- Improperly cleaning or maintaining a hair addition. Or getting poor advice on maintenance from an inexperienced specialist.

- Keeping a unit too long. Although some custom salons claim that a hair addition can last three or more years, no one will guarantee its actual appearance over that period. A more likely estimate is 18 to 24 months.

- Buying only one hair addition and not giving it up for repairs or maintenance. By wearing two or more hair additions in rotation, you can keep them both in good condition and delay each one's replacement up to 12 months or so.

eter. A technician pulls your growing hair up through the holes in the web and anchors the webbing to your scalp by sewing it to your hair. He or she weaves or sews wefts of artificial hair (human or synthetic) onto the anchored webbing. Another method of attaching the replacement wefts uses "tracks" of thread with multiple loops slightly raised above the webbing's surface. The technician attaches the wefts to each loop, gradually building up a full head of hair.

The cost of hair integration depends on where you have it done, but you can expect to pay up to $200 for your two-hour first visit and $50 to $75 each time you return to your salon for "maintenance." Your greatest expense will be maintaining this hair addition. Because your own anchoring hair continues to grow out, the replacement hair eventually lifts away from your scalp. Depending on how fast your hair grows, you have to visit your salon every four to eight weeks to have the addition retightened and your own hair cut and styled. Because of breakage or normal wear and tear, the entire integration may have to be redone every 18 months or so — for another $200 to $300.

Hair integration has certain advantages. If you're dissatisfied with the results, your stylist can remove it at any time. Assuming the salon has done a professional job, you can swim or exercise without fear of the integration unit coming loose or falling off. Also, the artificial hair is virtually undetectable, as long as the salon properly matches its color and texture to your own hair and then trims and styles your hair to achieve a proper blend.

Unfortunately, hair integration also has some drawbacks. It is complex and it requires special skill to produce good results. Because it requires regular visits to a salon equipped to handle it, your flexibility is limited—especially if you travel frequently. Shampooing and caring for your scalp and growing hair under the integration unit are also a problem. You must clean thoroughly to avoid buildup of bacteria and oils from the scalp while being careful not to break or loosen threads and webbing. You must use only wide-toothed combs or brushes and avoid striking the webbing and thread. Finally, the tight braiding or binding of your natural hair can cause further hair loss because of breakage or traction alopecia—a form of baldness that occurs when hair is under continuous tension.

Bonding — Bonding, like hair integration, works only on thinning hair. It doesn't work on a completely bald scalp because it requires gluing replacement hair to what you already have. A salon first matches the color of your remaining hair with "wefts" of human or synthetic hair. The stylist lifts and sections the naturally growing hair. He then applies a skin-compatible, polymer glue to one of these sections and to a weft of new hair. By

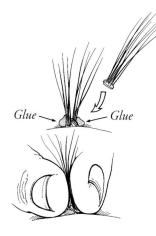

Glue — — Glue

Fig. 5-8. Gluing a weft of new hair to a section of naturally growing hair.

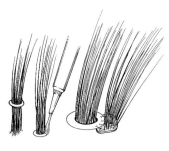

Fig. 5-9. Sewing wefts of replacement hair to nylon ringlets.

pressing these two sections together, he allows the glue to "fuse" them into place (fig. 5-8).

Or, the stylist will slide little nylon ringlets over the sections of growing hair and push them down to the scalp. He applies the polymer glue to each nylon ringlet and glues the ringlet to the base of each hair section. Using a fine nylon thread, he can sew the wefts of replacement hair to these nylon ringlets, blending them in with the growing hair (fig. 5-9).

By repeating either of these procedures on a number of sections, experienced stylists can quickly build up a full head of hair. They can also add frosted highlights or varying colors to slightly change your appearance. The process takes 30 to 45 minutes. After it's done, you can safely swim, exercise, and even color your hair.

The first bonding session can cost up to $200, with rebonding and styling recommended every 4 to 6 weeks. These regular applications, which run about $65 each, are necessary because your own hair continues to grow and because oils and pollutants affect the bonding agent. Thus, bonding could cost you just over $1,000 for the first year and about $800 per year from then on. If you're in your 30s when you begin, you could spend well over $25,000 before retirement age.

Besides the cost, maintenance is also a disadvantage with bonding. As with hair integration, you may find it inconvenient to visit a salon up to 13 times a year for rebonding sessions. Because fewer salons do this process, frequent travelers have special problems finding service away from home. In addition, you must shampoo bonded hair carefully, wash your hair only once every three to four days, use only wide-toothed combs and brushes, and avoid putting oils of any kind on your hair to prevent breaking down the bonds.

Individual Hair Implants

Although hair implants were popular in the 70s and 80s, after numerous complaints and lawsuits, the Food and Drug Administration banned them in the United

States. Even when implants were legal, the procedure was often done in "clinics" without proper medical supervision. These clinics frequently moved from city to city, staying one step ahead of legal action. We mention them here as a warning because you could run across a "bootleg" operation.

Implants were promoted as a "permanent" solution to baldness, an end to the costly maintenance and replacement of wigs or hair additions. Synthetic, hairlike fibers were injected or "implanted" directly into the scalp — either singly or in groups. A small knot or hook at the bottom of each fiber held the implant in place. An alternate method used human hair with its cuticle, or outer surface, stripped away. The idea was that a "pure" hair strand would be less likely to be rejected by the scalp as a foreign substance, so it wouldn't cause infection.

Despite claims that implants did not cause infection, many complications occurred from both kinds of hair implants. Infections often set in because any foreign material inserted into the scalp becomes a focus for the body's defense mechanism. In many cases, the only way to stop the infection was to remove the implants forcibly with tweezers or forceps. Removal caused severe pain, a psychological setback for the patient, and often, permanent scarring.

Among patients who didn't experience infection or inflammation, physicians reported many whose implanted hair began to fall out in irregular patches after 18 months or less. Many lost nearly all of the fiber implants within 10 weeks, and as much as 50 percent of the natural hair implants within three to four months. In some cases, the natural hair implants broke off at the surface of the scalp, leaving a short stubble that often caused severe infection. The implants were hard to remove, and patients suffered persistent pain and scarring. Needless to say, we don't consider hair implants an acceptable option. Working with a concerned state assemblyman, Mr. Michael Roos, we were able to pass legislation that made this procedure illegal in California.

Prostheses or Wigs

If someone loses all of his scalp hair, such as from chemotherapy or Alopecia Universalis — or Alopecia Totalis (all body hair), neither a hair addition nor hair surgery can help. There is no hair to transfer through surgery and no hair to anchor or complement a hair addition. The only solution is a wig or prosthesis to cover the entire head.

Wigs can be ready made or custom made, often with the same materials used in hair additions. They are usually less comfortable and may be less natural-looking than a hair addition, because they are replacing 22 to 24 inches of hairline. The neckline and areas around the ears are particularly difficult to conceal, and shorter hairstyles add to these difficulties. Fit is critical because full wig caps tend to ride up in the back on an active wearer.

Hair Additions Combined with Surgery

If you don't have enough donor hair for successful hair replacement surgery, you may be able to combine limited surgery with a hair addition to get better results. A common practice is to use hair grafts or a flap for a front hairline and then to place a hair addition behind the hairline for fuller coverage.

One of the most challenging parts of an ideal hair addition is establishing a natural hairline. On the sides and back of the head, a hair addition can be blended into the surrounding hair, but the hairline doesn't allow this blending. A hair transplant or rotation flap allows you to have your own hair at the hairline, to which your stylist can attach a hair addition for a natural look.

The disadvantage of this approach is that you can never go without the hair addition because you'll have hair only at the hairline and a horseshoe pattern of baldness behind it. Without the hair addition, you won't have a natural look. You would also be unable to go without a hairpiece later in life because the flap or transplants can't be removed without leaving some scarring that would no longer be covered by the growing hair.

If you can have complete hair-replacement surgery, you may wish to wear a hair addition while "under construction," although this is usually not necessary. Hair additions can make excellent cosmetic cover-ups between hair grafting procedures or scalp reductions.

In Summary

Hair additions can be a satisfactory alternative to hair loss for those who prefer not to undergo surgery or who are unqualified for it. If you can adjust to the fact that a hair addition is not your own hair, you can be very pleased with this option. Some people even like the fact that an addition isn't permanent. If they later decide to discontinue using it and to "grow old gracefully," they can. Also, if you're young and don't know how far your thinning may go, a hair addition is a reasonable option while you're waiting to decide about surgery.

Still, despite thousands of satisfied customers who have had their baldness covered with replacement hair, you may feel that wearing a hair addition is wrong for you. Some people are self-conscious about how an addition looks — even an expensive one. They're concerned that others will know they wear a hair addition and assert that they couldn't wear one without constantly adjusting it or looking in the mirror.

Although modern attachment techniques secure hair additions against the wind, most people wearing them still must be careful about playing certain sports or swimming. The oxidizing effects of chlorine and sun quickly cause a hair addition's color to contrast with the growing hair. Also, letting people run their fingers through an addition is risky at best—no replacement unit will stand up to vigorous "tousling" without being discovered.

Then too, you may find the cost and bother of hair additions impossible to bear. After all, if you're in your 30s when you start wearing them, you can spend $60,000 by the time you reach retirement age. And all the while you'd have to put up with tapes or glue, salon visits for maintenance, and extra problems with cleanliness and daily care.

If hair additions don't meet your needs, you'll want to know how to have your own hair growing on your own head permanently. The next chapter starts us in that direction by considering the potential for drugs and other medical treatments to eliminate hair loss.

6.
Other Non-surgical Approaches

The key to hair regrowth for balding people is to grow and keep enough terminal (normal) hairs to improve their appearance. Lotions or other techniques to stimulate hair growth must therefore restore this kind of hair to be effective.

To date, however, only minoxidil is approved by the Food and Drug Administration (FDA) for sale as a treatment for baldness. That means the FDA believes enough objective evidence exists to show that minoxidil can regrow some visible hair on some people. We'll say more about it, as well as a few other experimental treatments that may eventually prove they can grow some hair on bald scalp, in the next chapter.

For now, we'd like you to know about the most common "treatments" that have captured attention, and millions of dollars, from balding people throughout the world. We won't try to cover these products by name because new ones keep appearing all the time. But we can tell you they are usually based on one of three major theories for curing baldness:

- unclogging hair follicles
- increasing blood flow to the scalp
- improving the diet so more nutrients are available for hair growth

Once you've seen how these products claim to regrow hair, you should be able to read any company's literature and understand why they can't solve your male pattern baldness.

Unclogging Hair Follicles

Before we begin describing several "treatments" based on cleansing blocked hair follicles, we should point out that clogged follicles have nothing to do with male pattern baldness. Blockage of pores would cause sores to develop on the scalp, the way acne sores appear on faces that are excessively oily. Yet, most bald people have no problems of this kind. Also, as the beards of young adults demonstrate, oily skin itself has no effect on hair growth. Of course, as mentioned in Chapter Two, you may lose some hair temporarily if seborrhea develops from an oily, inflamed scalp. Untreated cases rarely may even lead to permanent loss of hair.

Other than these rare cases, the FDA and the medical community certainly don't accept the idea of permanent hair loss because of excess sebum--another way of saying that hair follicles are clogged. Studies show there's no difference in sebum levels between bald and non-bald men. In fact, some doctors believe the scalps of bald men may be less oily than those who have hair because the oil glands shrink along with the follicles during the balding process.

Despite scientific proofs to the contrary, a number of companies claim to be able to stop hair loss and even regrow hair by cleansing your follicles or controlling sebum production--and therefore releasing the trapped hair. Although this approach may sound logical, medical science has shown that cleaning your hair regularly can guard against hair loss from environmental damage but not from male pattern baldness. Some companies even claim that your blocked hair continues to grow underneath the scalp--up to eight inches long--and that it pops up like a spring once the scalp is cleaned with their herbal solutions. Again, we've never discovered hair of this type growing under the scalp, despite our surgical experience with thousands of bald patients.

The steps required to apply these solutions are also time-consuming. Often, you must spray a little "special" shampoo onto your scalp, wait from five to 30 minutes, and then massage in the formula for 20 to 30 minutes with a vibrator. After leaving the formula on for 24 hours, you start again. You must continue this treatment for nine to 18 months before you can get your money back if it fails.

These shampoos or solutions can cost up to $200 a month. They are often backed up by guarantees: "Your hair back or your money back." Unfortunately, you usually get only your last payment back, so if you were paying by the month, all but your last month's payment would be lost. If you pay for a several-month program in advance, you're often "covered" for the full amount, but you must use the formulas every night for the entire period. Stopping early would cancel the guarantee.

Polysorbate — This substance has been one of the biggest sellers ever in the over-the-counter market for hair restorers--millions of dollars worth in recent years. One reason polysorbate has been so successful may be that companies have pitched it as a scientific treatment. In 1978, Setala and Schreck-Purola published a paper describing their treatment of baldness with polysorbate 60. While doing cancer research in the pathology department at the University of Helsinki, Finland, they observed a side-effect from the solution used to move medication through the skin of rats: polysorbate 60 caused a faster regrowth of hair.

After further testing with animals, they tried polysorbate on the heads of bald men. They said their data showed new hair growth in about 60 percent of the patients and a higher percentage who saw their hair loss slow down considerably or stop. Soon, others began to market polysorbate treatments commercially in Europe and the United States. National advertisements quoting the scientific research and many testimonials boosted the acclaim of polysorbate 60 as a treatment for baldness.

Today, several companies offer polysorbate-based hair treatments, usually with advertisements referring to the Helsinki research. Some add biotin, niacin, cystine, or other products supposed to help hair grow. Of course, they don't actually claim to have a cure for baldness, because a baldness cure would have to be approved as a drug by the Food and Drug Administration. Instead, they claim to unclog your hair follicles, so hair can grow naturally.

Product literature explains the action of polysorbate as similar to the emulsifiers in floor cleaners which cut through "waxy buildup" and allow you to clean away the deep dirt below the wax surface. Supposedly, it emulsifies the "invisible film of DHT cholesterol" which edges into the hair follicle and forces your growing hair to become thinner and thinner as it "competes for space." Removing this "killer DHT" allows the besieged hair to reassert itself.

Unfortunately, this miracle substance found in many common products doesn't restore hair. The scientific research mentioned above was flawed for two reasons. The test involved 320 adults, but only 24 actually received the polysorbate and some of the patients didn't always come to have their hair growth checked during the trials. Also, the study was "uncontrolled." No other identical group (control group) received a placebo to see if results may have been from other factors.

An interview with the doctors who conducted the original study of polysorbate finally revealed that they had never claimed it was a cure for baldness. Instead, they believed it might slow the rate of balding and, in a few cases, stop excessive hair loss. Of course, hair loss in men is so variable that the role of a topical preparation like polysorbate is difficult to establish. A stabilizing period often follows rapid loss. After a few years, the loss might start up again. Thus, a man using polysorbate while rapidly losing his hair could coincidentally stabilize after taking it. If his loss began again later, he would think polysorbate stopped it temporarily.

An objective study of polysorbate 60 in 1985 showed no significant difference in hair growth among men who used it versus those who used only glycerine and water. All 174 men in this study were diagnosed as having male pattern baldness, and the procedure was "double-blind": researchers and subjects alike didn't know who was receiving polysorbate or glycerine and water. Still, about one in five men using the glycerine solution thought they had grown new hair--perhaps because glycerine makes hair appear thicker.

This perception explains why so many formulas can garner testimonials from "satisfied customers." People who experienced regrowth may have done so for another reason or simply thought they had new hair. Hope alone can exaggerate a bald person's perception of growth, but simply growing a bit of "peach fuzz" isn't enough to improve your appearance.

For a few ounces of polysorbate and distilled water, plus a like amount of shampoo, you can pay up to $50. Most companies consider this a 90-day supply. Some offer a money-back guarantee, but marketing research studies show that fewer than 10 percent of customers take companies up on these guarantees. Most of the other 90 percent either allow the time limit on the guarantee to expire or are reluctant to admit they've paid for something that doesn't reverse their hair loss.

Increasing Blood Flow to the Scalp

These "cures" do have some basis in fact, because a poor supply of blood can cause cell damage — and resulting hair loss — in the scalp. But this problem would exist only in cases of severe disease or severing of arteries and veins through injury. Many years of experience with transplant surgery have shown us that bald men have plenty of blood flow to support hair growth.

A related theory claims that baldness derives from having a thick galea (underlayer of the scalp) which blocks blood and nutrients from your follicles. But this idea flies in the face of an established medical fact:

there's no difference in the thickness of the galea in bald and non-bald men. Thus, as far as we can determine from experience and medical research, treatments based on either of these theories are unnecessary and ineffective for balding men.

Creams, Shampoos, and Massage — Creams or shampoos that claim to increase blood circulation in the scalp are often called hair regenerators, which are supposed to work by improving vasodilation--the dilation of small blood vessels. Some are recommended along with massage, which is often claimed to stimulate blood flow and therefore bring more nutrients to the hair follicles.

As we've mentioned previously, shampooing is good for your hair, but you can do it quite well at home with many fine products. At the same time, although massage may feel good and probably won't harm your hair (unless you pull and tangle it), there's no evidence that massage can permanently regrow lost hair. Stimulation of the scalp may produce some temporary growth of vellus hair, but no bald person we know of has had cosmetically significant growth from these techniques.

Galeal Thinners — Often made of amino acids and proteins, these formulas are supposed to thin the galea, allowing more blood to the follicles and thereby regrowing hair. Some companies claim to have seen a significant, observable increase in terminal (permanent) hair at the end of six months. But the lack of independent studies confirming results is suspicious, especially given the market for a truly effective cure. And, as we've mentioned, these shampoos or creams are based on an incorrect assumption about galeal thickness in bald scalps, which shows no average variation from people with full heads of hair.

To use formulas for increasing blood circulation or thinning your galea, you can pay $35-$75 a month, often without money-back guarantees. You must rub them into your scalp as often as twice a day and, in many cases, must wear heat caps or use vibrators on your scalp for 15-20 minutes with each application. Thus, you could easily spend $700 and 200 hours per year on a technique that has no proven effect on bald scalp.

Mechanical and Electrical Devices — Nearly 60 years ago, a man wrote to Scientific American that wearing a hat tightly over the temporal bones causes most pattern baldness. He insisted that the hat presses against and shrinks the arteries supplying blood to the scalp, causing the hair to die for want of blood. To cure his problem, this man underwent treatments which brought the blood back through these shrunken arteries to his hair roots by applying the ultra-violet rays of a mercury-vapor quartz lamp. These rays supposedly drew blood to the surface of the scalp, enlarged the arteries, and let more blood through to nourish the hair follicles, thus regrowing lost hair.

Although we may smile at the "primitive science" of the 1930s, trying to reverse baldness with electrical fields continues in at least two forms. One version is "hair popping," which uses a high-frequency machine to pass an electrical current through the body of a balding person holding a "saturator," or metal rod. The machine's operator then grabs the person's hair and lightly yanks it, completing an electrical circuit and giving the scalp a mild shock ("popping").

We're not sure if anyone in the United States is using this technique, but it is available in England and Europe at up to $600 for a series of 6 "pops." It depends on the fact that an electrical stimulus momentarily increases circulation of blood to the scalp, which is supposed to slow or prevent balding by improving nourishment of the hair follicle. We've already mentioned that, in our experience, balding men have normal blood circulation and are unlikely to need any special stimulation of the scalp. We also recommend against popping because it may cause traumatic hair loss from shock.

A second version of electrical treatment is undergoing tests. This method uses four pairs of positively and negatively charged electrodes connected to a 12-volt

Fig. 6-1. The Evans Vacuum Cap. One of many historical devices supposed to stimulate blood flow to bald scalp, thus improving nutrition to the hair follicles and causing hair to grow.

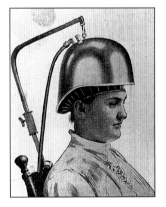

battery and placed within hoods similar to those in hair salons. Balding patients sit under the hoods and have their heads bathed in an electrical field. Unlike the current used in hair popping, this field causes no sensation in the scalp.

Based on a study of 50 balding men in 1990, "electrical baths" seemed to show some promise under limited circumstances. Researchers point out that it works only for people who have been bald for a short time and who retain their hair roots. It also must be continued to remain effective. It seems to stimulate dying hair follicles to produce DNA, the basic building block of human cells, which then develops into protein and hair synthesis. Researchers are uncertain how blood flow, electrical triggering, or other factors interact to create hair growth. Even if the technique proves to be effective, full use is still years away.

Improving Diet and Nutrition

Another common theory suggests that deficiencies in your diet can cause baldness and that you can regrow this lost hair by consuming certain foods. Some companies are marketing vitamins formulated specifically to help hair grow. These formulas usually contain Vitamin C, Inositol, PABA, L-Cysteine, and Biotin. Each of these vitamins has some connection to hair growth. PABA may reverse premature graying. L-Cysteine makes up 10 percent of your hair and, especially when combined with Vitamin C to keep it more soluble, has increased hair growth in animals. Taking them won't harm you, but few people suffer deficiencies that have an actual effect on hair loss. And no scientific evidence exists to show that eating special combinations of food or vitamins can grow hair on bald scalp.

As we mentioned earlier, a proper balance of fats, carbohydrates, and proteins is necessary for healthy hair growth. Deficiencies in your diet can cause temporary hair loss--usually reversible with a change in eating habits. Unfortunately, nutrition has nothing to do with male-pattern baldness. If you eat a normal, reasonably balanced diet, your hair will receive all the nutrients it needs for growth. In fact, according to research studies, even the starving in developing countries and survivors from concentration camps during World War II showed little difference in rates of baldness compared to people on normal diets. At the same time, if your hair is programmed to fall out, no evidence exists to suggest that nutritional "treatments" can stop or restore it. Because this kind of programmed loss is responsible for 95 percent of the hair loss in balding men, we caution you against such miracle diets.

Nutriol — According to its official distributor in the United States, Nutriol is a cosmetic that gives your hair a fuller appearance but doesn't help baldness. But the same Nutriol is marketed in other countries as a baldness treatment. In the United States, Nutriol is now marketed as a hair care "system" to make your hair look and feel good. As a hair care product, Nutriol seems to us rather expensive. Many fine shampoos and conditioners are available at a fraction of the cost. As long as you don't expect it to reverse your baldness, it is up to you to decide whether it is worth the money.

Biotin — A popular type of nutritional scalp formula incorporates biotin, a B-complex vitamin, as its major ingredient. Our bodies don't manufacture their own supply of biotin because we get plenty of it from our diets or from bacteria living in our intestines. If we ate only egg whites or received intravenous feedings for extended periods, we might have a biotin deficiency that causes hair loss. Otherwise, with few exceptions, we don't need biotin supplements.

Research cited by purveyors of biotin formulas to show that it has regrown hair has not involved male pattern baldness. Usually, studies deal with alopecia areata, or patchy baldness, which may respond to cortisone and other treatments as well as to biotin. Yet, biotin has become a very popular ingredient in creams and tonics claiming to restore hair. Its supporters believe biotin

Fig. 6-2. Benton's Hair Grower. A historical potion which claimed to "fertilize" the scalp and promote natural hair growth. Dozens of similar creams have been sold to deep-clean or stimulate bald scalp to produce hair.

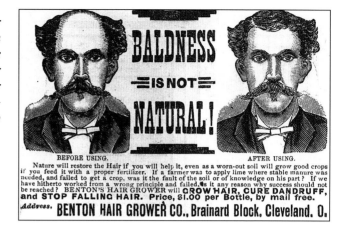

binds testosterone in the hair follicle instead of allowing the testosterone to bind with the protein receptors that turn it into DHT. Because less DHT is available to "attack" the follicle, hair loss supposedly slows down or stops.

To use biotin formulas, you typically must apply biotonic conditioner once a day and pat a lotion or cream into your scalp nightly. In some cases, companies recommend biotonic hair sprays for extra body in styling. They claim you should see an end to your hair fall after eight to 10 weeks and hair growth after 10 to 18 weeks of continuous treatment. Some "clinics" recommend an office visit to start the program, a full line of products, and twice monthly "checkups" in the early stages. If you were to buy the full treatment lasting some 18 months, you could spend up to $2,000. After that, you must continue to use the products to maintain your results.

The Food and Drug Administration denies the effectiveness of biotin in slowing the balding process. Independent studies of biotin formulas have found no significant difference in the amount of hair loss between those receiving the biotin and those in control groups. We consider biotin programs an expensive way to care for your hair.

Hair Analysis — Hair analysis is often linked with nutritional "cures" for baldness, because your hair reflects the amount of certain minerals, metals, and toxic substances you've consumed. The procedure consists of taking hair samples and subjecting them to chemical tests on an atomic absorption spectrophotometer, which can analyze their content. Scientific literature does reveal some legitimate uses for this technique. For example, diabetics are deficient in chromium--a correlation that may lead to treatment. Copper level changes may be linked to liver problems. And sodium levels are up to five times normal in people who have cystic fibrosis. Other deficiencies in trace elements may be an early warning sign for esophagus cancer. Recently, companies and government agencies have employed hair analysis to test employees' use of amphetamines and barbiturates, which may show up in your hair even when they're undetectable in the blood.

Unfortunately, these discoveries have led to unscrupulous "hawking" of hair analysis as the solution for hair loss. All you have to do, the advertisements say, is to discover the nutritional cause of your loss by analyzing what is missing or deficient in your hair. Then, you can purchase vitamin and mineral supplements that will reverse your balding or cure various other ailments.

As the Food and Drug Administration has proved, however, we simply can't take your hair sent in a bag and tell you what your nutritional status is. For one thing, hair analysis can't tell us anything about your vitamin intake. Also, minerals in your hair may not closely match those in your diet or blood, because the environment, smoking, drinking alcohol, and seasonal changes can affect your hair at any given time.

Basically, hair is dead protein (see Chapter One), so it can't reveal what a sample of living tissue can about your health. Together with detailed information about your age, diet, drug intake, smoking or drinking habits, occupation, and use of hair products, hair analysis at a legitimate laboratory can back up other tests. But you should be aware that people have sent hair from their dogs to mail-order analysis companies and received a detailed report about their future baldness and how to prevent it.

Are Over-the-Counter Approaches for You?

If these approaches don't work, you're probably wondering what explains their marketing success. Despite the Food and Drug Administration's ban on advertising these treatments as hair restorers, you may still see claims of dramatic hair growth on balding men and women. In some cases, you may even read testimonials from satisfied customers and see wonderful "before and after" photographs of this growth. These compelling advertisements can easily capture the attention of someone who is seeking a cure for his hair loss.

You must use special caution when evaluating before and after photographs of hair loss and restoration. Because of variations in lighting and positioning, they may mask the true result. Very careful photographic technique is necessary to accurately show the effects of a baldness treatment.

Logically, we understand that a true, safe hair restorative wouldn't need a single dollar for marketing or advertisement. Within weeks it would be a multi-billion-dollar product, purchased by joyful bald men throughout the world. Unfortunately, no such product exists. If you want a full head of your own hair or cosmetically significant regrowth, we don't know of any non-prescription treatment that can provide it. In the next chapter, we discuss prescription preparations that offer slight rays of hope a solution may someday appear.

7.
Prescription Drugs Under Development

Prescription preparations may eventually be a promising source of non-surgical treatment for baldness, but present results are tentative, and all of the preparations mentioned in this chapter except Rogaine are years away from potential approval by the FDA as hair restoratives. Still, some interesting investigation is under way on drugs that affect blood flow to the scalp, combat the effects of male hormones on hair cells, regulate immune-system reactions against hair follicles, and alter the genetic coding for hair loss.

Minoxidil and Its Variants

While other drugs undergo painstaking development, only Upjohn's minoxidil (Rogaine) enjoys FDA approval for sale to balding patients with a physician's prescription. It began as a licensed treatment for high blood pressure, but hair growth on bald scalps (as well as some unwanted locations) appeared as a side-effect. Because it was already approved by the FDA to treat high blood pressure, doctors were initially able to prescribe it as a treatment for baldness--usually by having pharmacists crush tablets and mix them in a solution for topical application. Patients then rubbed the solution on their scalps twice each day.

After more than a decade of testing, minoxidil finally appeared on the market as Rogaine in 1988. Recent television advertisements and a $50 million annual advertising budget began to pay off during 1990, resulting in sales of some $175 million. Upjohn considers Rogaine a disappointment compared to their original estimates of $500 million in annual sales. But it has done well considering its actual effectiveness and FDA restrictions on advertising, which disallow descriptions of its properties without a full list of side-effects and complications.

Although early studies suggested that minoxidil could regrow some hair on up to 30 percent of bald crowns (back of the head), our own experience with the drug was not quite as successful as we had initially hoped for. According to some physicians, it is more effective in cutting the rate of hair loss among young men whose loss is recent. They report that a high percentage of young men using Rogaine will start slowing the balding process within two months of the first application. Our experience with Rogaine has shown that relatively few young men can slow down hair loss temporarily. Patients have reported that this slowdown lasts about 12 to 18 months, and sometimes a little longer. But balding resumes if a person stops using Rogaine.

Even before Upjohn released Rogaine, researchers were looking for ways to improve minoxidil's performance. For example, one doctor developed a product that he felt was much more effective than minoxidil alone. He claimed 70 to 90 percent of his patients got good results. His ingredients included a "DHT blocker" that he said was responsible for its increased effectiveness when compared to minoxidil. No independent studies have confirmed whether this product performs as claimed. If the DHT blocker were effective, it could give better results than minoxidil alone, but the only DHT blockers available are very weak and for the most part ineffective. In any case, this product costs more than Rogaine and also has to be used for a lifetime to maintain the regrowth of hair.

More recently, some physicians have added Retin-A

to Rogaine, which seems to increase absorption of minoxidil into the scalp and may make it more effective. Unfortunately, minoxidil's varying rate of effectiveness, tendency to help younger men with crown baldness, cost (about $75 per month), and requirement for twice-a-day applications throughout one's lifetime to avoid losing regrown hair all make it much less than a perfect solution for baldness. This may explain why it has not become as popular as we originally anticipated.

Combatting Male Hormones

Because male hormones are a prime element in balding, many researchers have concentrated on reducing the level of these hormones in the scalp. Though correct in theory, a safe treatment has been difficult to find. In 1988, Dr. Marty Sawaya isolated three forms of protein in scalp tissue that may be the keys to finding a cure. Two are receptors for testosterone. Active hair follicles contain nearly equal amounts of both proteins, but follicles from bald scalp contain two times as much of the smaller protein--the one associated with baldness.

Perhaps even more important was Sawaya's discovery of a third protein which suppresses the amount of testosterone binding to the smaller protein mentioned above. This "inhibitor protein" prevents buildup of male hormones and their eventual conversion to DHT--the substance that triggers genetically programmed follicles to stop producing hair. Work is now under way to purify this inhibitor protein and use it to develop an antibody against the protein receptor that causes hair loss. Meanwhile, several other drugs are under development as baldness treatments based on their ability to inhibit the effects of male hormones on hair follicles.

Progesterone — Thirty years ago, researchers already knew that the female hormone, progesterone, would bind with an enzyme in the hair follicles (5-alpha reductase) which converts normal testosterone into DHT (dihydrotestosterone). As we've pointed out, DHT combines with protein receptors in hair follicles programmed for baldness and causes the hair to fall out. But progesterone removes much of the available enzyme and, therefore, the DHT that must be present for baldness to occur. Unfortunately, if a balding man ingests enough progesterone to slow his hair loss, he can take on feminine characteristics (enlarged breasts, soft features, and so on). Given this choice, most men prefer to remain bald.

Theoretically, progesterone applied to the scalp might slow the rate of balding, but no clinical trials have proven that it does, and we've never seen any evidence of this effect. Also, topical progesterone would have to be used in small doses to be safe. Sadly, these doses are too small to cause your hair to regrow.

Because of potential side-effects, only a doctor can treat you with progesterone. Your doctor would either inject it directly into your scalp or prescribe an ointment, in a concentration of no more than two or four percent, which you would apply twice a day.

Anti-Androgens — Other treatments directed at fighting the balding effects of testosterone employ anti-androgens, such as cyproterone acetate, flutamide, or cyoctol. Like progesterone, anti-androgens may create feminine characteristics in men. Because of these side-effects, they may not be a cure for common male baldness on their own, but they have produced new information. Early trials by manufacturers suggest that anti-androgens can grow hair on bald scalp, but until we see further evidence of actual results, we have to consider them an experimental and distant solution.

Cyoctol has generated considerable interest within the last two years because of reports on early research and acquisition of its marketing rights by the Squibb Corporation. Chantal Pharmaceutical Corporation originally developed it as a treatment for acne. Both acne and hair loss are related to high levels of DHT near the skin's surface. Cyoctol counteracts the effects of DHT by binding to the hair follicle cells before they can bind to DHT and begin to die off.

Squibb released some preliminary results on a very small number of people at the end of 1989. Their trials showed hair growth in 10 of 12 men who rubbed a 0.5 percent cyoctol ointment on their scalps for 48 weeks. These men had an average gain of 40 hairs in a small balding area at the upper back area of their heads, whereas most men receiving a placebo solution lost an average of 65 hairs. In a 1990 follow-up study, 83 percent of the 32 men who used cyoctol for a year saw an average of 11 percent new hair growth in similar small areas on their crowns. Unfortunately, because of the small number of subjects in each trial, the results aren't statistically significant.

One encouraging sign is that cyoctol didn't enter the bloodstream of any volunteer, so it overcame the anti-androgens' common problem of causing female traits in men. But the ointment contained a relatively low percentage of the drug (one-fourth the concentration of commercially distributed minoxidil, or Rogaine). Researchers intend to continue testing at a higher dosage to see whether cyoctol becomes more effective--without damaging side-effects. They expect side-effects to be minimal because none have appeared in tests on animals at much higher concentrations.

As you might imagine, cyoctol's promise as a commercial preparation to treat baldness lies years in the future and depends on much more research with larger numbers of people. Until it clears the hurdles of further research, all-important FDA approval, and marketing in an economy laden with "cures" and disappointments, it is just another experimental candidate for hair restoration.

Other Future Treatments for Baldness

Rogaine has at least shown that some men can regrow some hair — even though the hair is gone, the follicles aren't dead. Following Upjohn's lead, Lederle Laboratories has had some interesting results with synthetic prostaglandin, a hormone-like substance normally produced by the body. Their drug based on this substance is called **Viprostol**. Like minoxidil, it acts as a vasodilator (relaxes the walls of blood vessels, thereby increasing the flow).

The results of an initial study on 150 men were encouraging, although a number of the men using Viprostol weren't helped at all. In a second scientific trial, conducted in 1990, tests on 57 men showed no hair growth after 6 months. Two observers counting new growth in photographs of the balding margin

HOW DO MEN FEEL ABOUT THEIR HAIR LOSS?

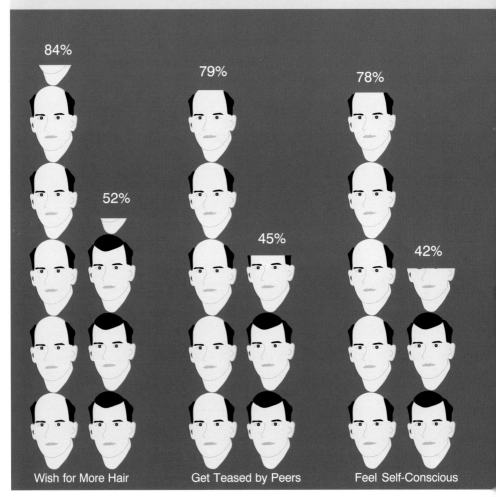

found that growth actually declined over the period. They also found no significant difference between an untreated group of men and the groups treated with a plain lotion or the lotion containing Viprostol. More testing will have to take place before results are conclusive. Because this drug doesn't have FDA approval for other applications, no one can prescribe it to treat male-pattern baldness until it's officially approved for this purpose.

Diazoxide, initially marketed as a treatment for

Psychological perceptions of male-pattern baldness — in society as a whole and among balding men themselves — have helped fuel a multi-billion dollar industry for prescription drugs and other non-surgical treatments. A recent survey by Dr. Thomas Cash, Professor of Psychology at Old Dominion University, shows that balding men are very sensitive about their condition. When compared to men with minimal hair loss, balding men in general feel self-conscious, less attractive, and even helpless about their hair loss.

= men with extensive hair loss.   = men with little or moderate hair loss.

56%

51%

37%

41%

31%

23%

Feel Helpless About MPB   Feel Less Attractive   Wear Hats or Caps hyperglycemia (too much sugar in the blood), may also have promise. Like minoxidil, it caused hair growth in unwanted areas when taken orally. If it were formulated as a solution and applied only to the scalp, some evidence shows that it might get hair to grow on bald heads.

In a recent study of diazoxide use by 25 human volunteers, 11 completed the study, and all grew some new hair. Several produced full-size terminal hairs. Consequently, researchers have asked the FDA for permission to test the effects of diazoxide on 400 volunteers.

Tricomin is another drug that may eventually be applied as a remedy for baldness, but its results so far are highly tentative and in need of confirmation by independent studies. Tricomin is a peptide-copper combination derived from a natural compound that triggers the body's mechanism for tissue repair. ProCyte, a biopharmaceutical company that focuses on tissue repair, discovered that Tricomin caused thick hair growth in mice. They then tested it on 18 men in France, where the regulatory process is faster. According to the company, those who got the strongest dose of Tricomin grew some hair, with no apparent side effects. ProCyte will need to do considerably more testing with larger numbers of people to prove Tricomin's effectiveness.

One last drug worth mentioning in the fight against baldness is **Proscar**, an anti-androgen developed by Merck Sharp and Dohme to treat enlarged prostates. It shrinks the prostate by blocking male hormones--the same hormones that convert testosterone to follicle-killing DHT in the balding process. Although Proscar has not been tested for effectiveness in restoring hair, Merck announced plans to begin testing in 1993. Even if it turns out to be successful, it wouldn't reach the market before the end of the century.

Immune-system research may be a new angle of attack on baldness. Researchers believe hair loss could be a result of your body's immune system setting up defenses against itself. Normally, your immune system keeps you safe from foreign cells, such as bacteria or viruses. It has "scout cells" that watch for and identify foreign "invaders," as well as "killer cells" that destroy the enemy cells and create antibodies. Memory cells remember what the invader looks like so future attacks can quickly be brought under control.

At times, though, your immune system gets mixed signals and views friendly cells as invaders. In the case of hair loss, DHT may provoke the immune system into action against "good" and "bad" protein receptors. Antibodies therefore would continue to attack hair follicles when hair tries to regrow.

Other researchers believe that antibodies are attacking hair pigment cells in your growing hair bulbs, thereby turning hair on your bald scalp fine and colorless. If so, your hair loss may just be a coincidental result of the attack on pigment cells. As reinforcement for this concept, researchers cite the case of a person losing only red hairs inherited from a redheaded father who went bald at 35. Because the person's black hair didn't fall out, they believe his antibodies may have been programmed against red pigment.

These complex interactions seem reasonable, but much more research is necessary before anyone can develop a treatment based on immune-system responses.

Further research on protein receptors and inhibitors, as well as work on gene splicing, may give us other approaches. We know that the genes for baldness and for hair color reside in the cells of each hair follicle rather than in the surrounding skin. Thus, if a young person's genetic message can be altered, either by altering the genes themselves or by readjusting the distribution of proteins in our scalps, we may never have to lose our hair. Some researchers even speculate we may someday have "gene creams"--topical preparations that, when rubbed into the scalp, will seep into the hair follicles and alter their genetic coding. Along with the anti-androgens described earlier, these experimental approaches may prove to be far better than minoxidil in counteracting various forms of baldness.

Research on prescription preparations holds promise. In fact, some doctors believe these preparations may eventually eliminate hair loss for millions of balding men. However, if you want to solve your baldness today, rather than waiting years for scientific breakthroughs, you must turn to the other alternatives discussed in the following chapters.

8.
Scalp Reductions

Although scalp reductions aren't useful on their own to solve male pattern baldness, we believe they are vital to managing baldness in almost every patient undergoing punch grafting or flap procedures (discussed in Chapters 9 and 10). We want to explain the advantages of scalp reduction and comment on when you shouldn't have such surgery. We'll also discuss various ways of doing reduction incisions, describe the procedure in detail, and tell you about possible complications and their treatment.

With scalp reductions, we surgically remove parts of the bald skin and then stretch the surrounding hair-bearing scalp to close the defect in the area from which the bald skin was removed. In this way we not only decrease the bald area but also increase the size of the donor scalp area (fig. 8-1). By reducing a patient's bald scalp, we now have a smaller bald area to treat with transplants or flaps. In patients who are borderline candidates for hair-replacement surgery because they have a relatively small donor area, reductions may improve the chances of obtaining a good result. The success of hair-replacement surgery depends on the rule of "supply and demand" — how big is the bald area relative to the donor scalp.

Scalp reductions are also effective for removing burned or scarred scalp. If the scalp has enough elastic-

Fig. 8-1. As we remove bald skin with scalp reduction surgery, the size of the donor scalp increases. (1) Donor hair before reduction. (2, 3, and 4) Progressive increase in size of donor area after first, second, and third scalp reductions.

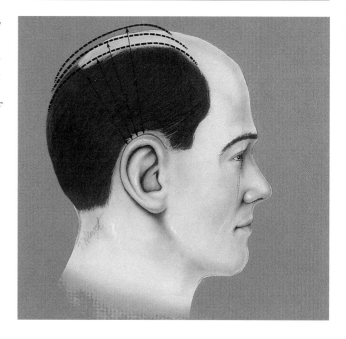

ity, we can do one or more reductions to remove this skin, as discussed further in Chapter 14 on reconstructive surgery.

Scalp-Reduction Patterns

If you talk to surgeons about scalp reduction, you'll discover differences in the patterns they use to decrease your baldness. Being aware of each pattern's advantages and disadvantages will allow you to choose a surgeon and a procedure that meet your expectations. We believe the goal of scalp reduction surgery is to remove as much bald skin as possible with the fewest reductions, as long as we don't increase the risk of complications or length of the post-operative recovery.

Fig. 8-2. Midline Ellipse. Stippled area represents area of skin excision.

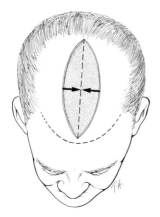

Midline Ellipse — The easiest and most common scalp-reduction pattern is the elliptic-midline closure (fig. 8-2). Many clinics use this procedure, which makes it easy to estimate the area of skin to be removed and causes no numbness of the scalp after the operation. Finally, the midline ellipse keeps blood flowing well from the lower part of your head to all parts of the scalp, whereas some incisions can block this flow and therefore create an area of scalp at the top of your head that has a poorer blood supply.

This midline pattern has significant disadvantages. For example, it isn't as good as other procedures because it removes bald skin only from side to side, whereas others also remove skin front to back. As a result, you're likely to need more reductions with the midline pattern to eliminate the same amount of baldness. Also, the midline pattern often distorts your remaining bald area, causing the back of your scalp to have an unnatural appearance. That's because the baldness in this area normally has a circular pattern, and the midline incision creates a slot or "axe-like" look (fig. 8-3). Therefore, we almost never use this pattern.

Lateral Pattern — Many surgeons use the lateral pattern of scalp reduction because of its advantages over the midline elliptical incision. The incision is on the side and rear of the head, nearer the border of growing hair, so the resulting scar isn't as visible as a mid-scalp scar (fig. 8-4). In addition, the surgeon can move more of the scalp forward from the back of the head with each reduction, eliminating more bald skin.

We seldom use the lateral pattern, however, because it distorts the remaining bald area as much as the midline pattern does. It also causes temporary numbness over the top of the head. Finally, it may create a central island of bald skin with reduced circulation. This occurs because the surgeon first does an incision on one side of the head and then goes back and does the other side. The two incisions cut off circulation from the lower part of the head, which can slow the growth of any grafts placed into that part of the scalp.

"Y" or "Double Y" Pattern — We've used these patterns in nearly all of our scalp reductions since 1977. As you can see in figures 8-5 and 8-6, we remove excess scalp front to back and side to side, thus taking out more bald skin than any other procedure does. Therefore, fewer reductions are necessary. The "Y" or "Double Y" also leaves a more natural hair growth in a circular pat-

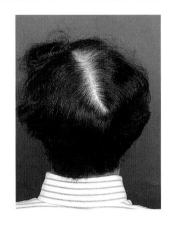

Fig. 8-3. Patient received a scalp reduction using the midline ellipse pattern before coming to our office. The midline incision created a slot or "axe-like" look by destroying the normal circular pattern within the crown. The hair grows in opposite directions and exposes a wide scar.

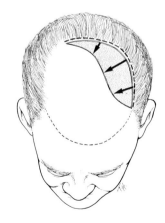

Fig. 8-4. Lateral Pattern. Stippled area represents area of skin excision.

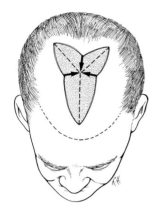

Fig. 8-5. Y pattern. Stippled area represents the excised skin.

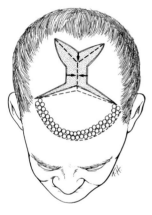

Fig. 8-6. Double Y pattern. This pattern prevents elevation of the recessions at the lateral sides of the hairline which would occur with the midline ellipse or Y patterns. With a Double Y pattern the location and curve of the hairline remains unchanged. Stippled area represents the excised skin.

tern away from the central bald area and avoids the central island of reduced circulation common to the lateral method.

If your bald scalp has an unusual shape, the "Y" or "Double Y" can adjust easily to it with simple variations in the length or angle of the "Y" incisions. In terms of cosmetic results, these patterns are especially impressive. They leave no scar on the middle back part of the head. Thus, if you had extensive baldness, we could leave the balding skin at the crown and still do a reduction in front of it.

The "Y" or "Double Y" pattern does have a few disadvantages, especially to the less experienced surgeon. It's technically more difficult than the midline ellipse and will probably take longer because more tissue is removed. It takes a bit more care in closing the incision to avoid excess scarring. It also might cause some cell damage at the tip of the flap that forms the "Y." But this has never happened in any of our patients, even though we close a reduction under moderate tension.

A "Double Y" incision is particularly effective if you've had grafting done on the front of your head, where we wouldn't want to raise the recessions at the junction of your temples and front hairline. In this case, we would place the limbs of the front "Y" behind the grafts, so we could stretch the hair at your temples without raising your hairline (fig. 8-7).

Procedure for Scalp Reductions

All hair-replacement procedures require care and skill but are safe and straightforward, with very few complications. Normally, you would have a scalp reduction under local anesthesia, but you can request intravenous or general anesthesia if you're especially anxious.

Typically, we cleanse your scalp with an antiseptic solution and then use an instrument called a Dermajet to place anesthesia into the surface of your scalp from one side of your head to the other. You may have heard that receiving local anesthesia is the most painful aspect

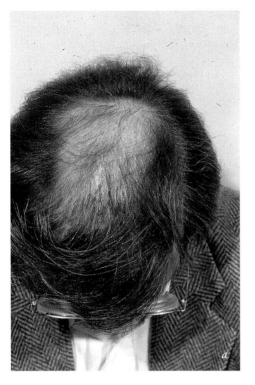 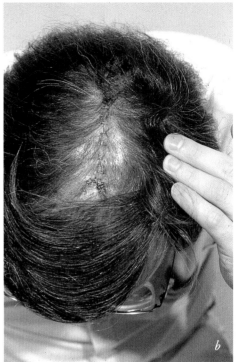

of scalp-reduction or hair-replacement surgery. But the Dermajet is a very gentle device; it makes subsequent injections virtually painless.

To numb your scalp completely, we follow the Dermajet with additional injections. In about 10 minutes, we can begin the surgery. We remove about one and a half to two inches of bald skin, depending on the elasticity of your scalp.

As a surgeon becomes more experienced, he can place more tension on the skin and remove larger amounts of baldness with each procedure. We've found that using more tension may lead to fewer reductions overall. After removing the excess skin, we close the incision and apply the dressings.

Any discomfort you have on the evening of surgery can be controlled with oral medication. You return the following morning for removal of your dressing. After the dressing is off, you may wash and blow dry your hair (usually on cooler settings) and return to work. About

Fig. 8-7a (above left). Appearance before scalp reductions but after punch grafts were placed at the hairline.

Fig. 8-7b (above right). Postoperative appearance after three reductions in a Double Y pattern. No elevation of the hairline occurred.

10 to 14 days after surgery, you'll have all sutures within the scalp removed--either in our office or, if you're from out of town or out of state, through other arrangements.

If you're going to have more than one scalp reduction, you would need to wait about 12 weeks before the next procedure. That's how long it takes for your scalp to return to its normal elasticity after a reduction.

Complications After Surgery

Fig. 8-8a (below left) and 8-8b (below right). Patient had a Y pattern scalp reduction. The posterior scalp has been advanced toward the front and the sides of the scalp elevated toward the top of the head which creates a more natural appearance of the crown than when midline incisions are made.

Scalp reductions have produced very few complications, and all have been minor. For example, pain is greater when we use more tension to close the reduction, but this enables us to remove more bald skin. The forehead could swell slightly, but we rarely see this swelling because of the medication given to all patients. Hematoma — a clotting or pooling of blood that causes swelling — almost never occurs and is easily solved. Infection is possible but extremely rare. If it occurs, we can treat it with antibiotics.

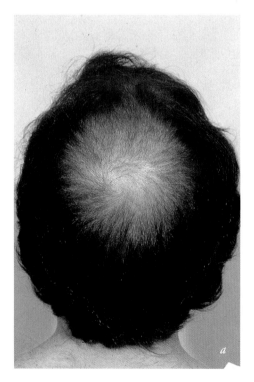
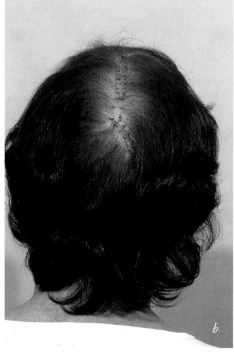

Cosmetic Problems After Surgery

Opposing Hair Direction — If your surgeon removes a lot of bald skin, your hair on each side of the incision could grow in opposite directions in the middle and back parts of your scalp, thus exposing a scar (fig. 8-3). Opposing hair direction is especially vexing with the midline incision because of the slot deformity mentioned earlier. The best way to correct this problem is to avoid it in the first place by not removing all fringe scalp along the suture line. By fringe scalp, we mean the area of your head with low-density hair between your bald skin and thicker hair. If your surgeon keeps some of your low-density hair in place, he can punch graft this area and direct some of the central grafts forward to help cover the scar. As we've already discussed, using a "Y" pattern partially prevents this problem because hair growth around the incision more naturally follows the crown (fig. 8-8).

Stretching of the Bald Scalp — The most tension in a scalp reduction is on tissue next to the incision. Therefore, in a midline reduction, the most stretch occurs in the adjacent bald skin, with a lesser amount in the hair-bearing (donor) area on the sides and back of the scalp. The bald scalp usually stretches about 10 to 20 percent, and some have reported it to be as much as 30 to 40 percent. In our experience, the smaller amount has been the case and is of little significance. With a lateral pattern of scalp reduction, the hair-bearing donor area next to the incision may stretch significantly. In this case, your hair density would decrease, so we rarely use this pattern.

Poor Healing of Incision Scars — We've never seen this problem in our patients, except in a rare patient with a history of bad scarring. Usually, with proper tension on the closure and the skin edges joined together carefully, you'll have no trouble with surgical scars. Of course, you must be aware that all scars remain red for several weeks before fading, so redness alone doesn't indicate poor healing.

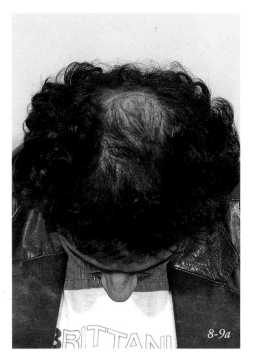

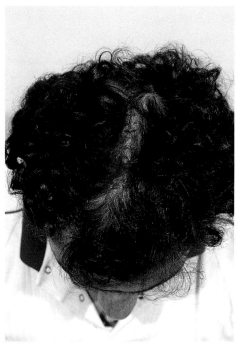

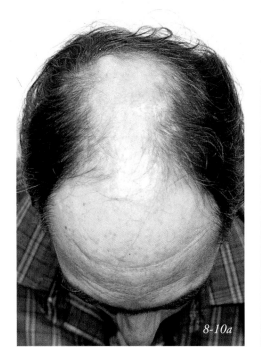

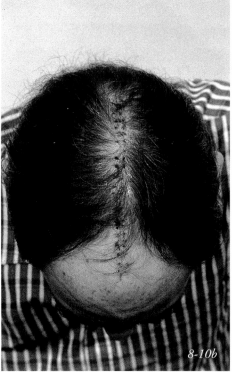

When You Shouldn't Have Scalp Reductions

Scalp reduction is most useful in scalps with the most elasticity, that is, scalps which wrinkle greatly when we push both sides up toward the top of your head. If you have a very tight scalp, you're not a good candidate for a scalp reduction, unless we do the reduction after tissue expansion (see Chapter 12). The gain you could get from reducing a tight scalp wouldn't be worth the time and expense. Fortunately, a small percentage of all people fall into this category.

We would not recommend a scalp reduction if you have only frontal hair loss and will never have further loss. If you're never going to have balding of the mid-scalp or crown, you don't need a scalp reduction. But if you're a young man with frontal loss, and your ultimate balding pattern will extend to your mid-scalp and crown, we usually go ahead with reductions before doing flaps (fig. 8-9). In fact, scalp reductions combined with flaps are the most effective way to treat baldness of the mid-scalp and crown while ensuring proper hair distribution throughout your lifetime (fig. 8-10).

Extensive Scalp Reductions (the Marzola procedure)

In 1984, Dr. Mario Marzola described a way to incise the scalp from near the temple along the fringe hairline to the back of the head. Bradshaw added to this method by doing both sides at the same time.

Thus, with what has come to be known as the Marzola-Bradshaw procedure, a surgeon can loosen and move forward the entire hairbearing scalp during a single reduction. He then completes the front hairline either by shifting a small hair flap from the upper part of the donor area or, in most cases, by punch grafting the midline and front of the scalp. Because you may run across this procedure while searching for hair-replacement techniques, we want to comment briefly on it.

An extensive reduction will remove much more of your bald mid-scalp and crown if your scalp has enough

Fig. 8-9a (opposite top left). Pre-operative view. Patient has only minimal hair loss at the hairline, but extensive loss within the center of his scalp (midscalp and crown).

Fig. 8-9b (opposite top right). Two reductions have virtually eliminated baldness at this time. Flaps or transplants will remove future baldness at the hairline.

Fig. 8-10a (opposite bottom left). Pre-operative view. Patient with Class III baldness.

Fig. 8-10b (opposite bottom right). Three scalp reductions have significantly reduced baldness of the crown and central scalp. The unimproved frontal baldness will require treatment with transplants or flaps.

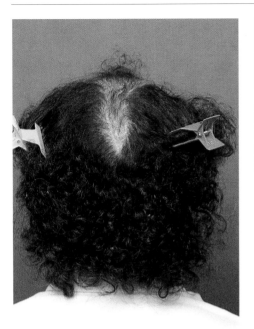

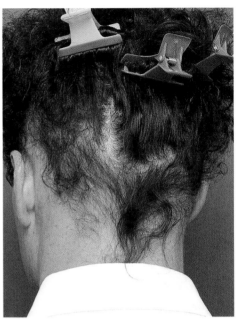

Fig. 8-11a (above left). Patient who had extensive scalp reductions before coming to us. Note the divergent thin hair growth and "axe-like" appearance in the mid-scalp and crown.

Fig. 8-11b (above right). Low-density hair at base of scalp has been stretched causing thinning and elevation in this part of scalp.

Fig. 8-11c (right). Scars along temporal hairline and into sideburns are difficult to conceal.

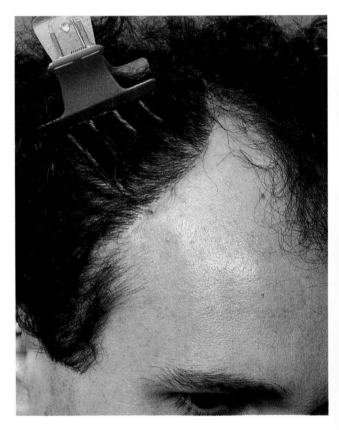

elasticity—but this is rare. Because an extensive reduction advances growing hair into the bald area, any stretching near the incision occurs within the hair-bearing area and not in the bald skin. Finally, this reduction increases the size of your donor area, so more donor hair is available. More donor hair means a surgeon can take more punch grafts from the increased donor area and transfer them to your front hairline. Added grafts will give your hairline more density, which results in a more natural look.

We have to accept some bad news, or disadvantages, along with these gains. Extensive reductions work only on highly elastic scalps and require much more anesthesia because the surgeon is operating over a larger area. They cause greater blood loss than normal reductions, present a special danger of losing scalp tissue to cell damage, and often cause hair loss in the stretched area as a result of poor circulation caused by too much tension. These reductions may also restrict neck motion if surgery pulls the skin at the nape of your neck too tight. Total numbness of your scalp at the back of your head and partial numbness at the temples and sides will continue up to one year after surgery.

In addition to these surgical limitations, extensive reductions also have some disadvantages to your appearance. They may cause considerable temporary loss of hair because of surgical shock (telogen effluvium). At the same time, they stretch the low-density ("scruffy") hair at the base of your neck and behind your ears, making that area appear even thinner. Divergent hair growth and a central scar after reduction make it impossible to get adequate height and density in your mid-scalp hair.

Another cosmetic defect from extensive reductions is a scar at the front of each temple which is difficult to conceal. As you get older, thinning or receding hair in this area will leave the scar more visible. Typically, you'll need further punch grafting to conceal these scars, and the results are often unsatisfactory. In such cases reconstructive surgery with scalp expansion may be necessary (fig. 8-11).

We believe this long list of disadvantages greatly outweighs the advantages of extensive scalp reductions. Conventional scalp reductions combined with punch grafting--discussed in the next chapter--will give you similar results. And, as you'll see in Chapter 10, scalp reductions together with flap surgery give you far superior results with less risk of serious complications. Standard scalp reductions, especially those using the more advanced incision patterns and procedures discussed in this chapter, have greatly improved the outcome of hair-replacement surgery.

9.
Transplants

Because transplanting (also called punch grafting) is easy for many doctors and technicians to do, it is the most common type of hair-replacement surgery. But it is also limited in its results. An average of 500-600 standard-sized punch grafts are available for transplanting—enough to cover frontal baldness but not enough to cover large bald areas (fig. 9-1). If you have or will have full male-pattern baldness, transplants can give you at best a moderately thinning appearance. Twenty years ago, you would have had to accept this limitation because punch grafting was the only surgical solution for lost hair. Today, scalp reductions, tissue expansion, and flap surgery give better results in most patients.

Once you're aware of the limitations of punch grafting, you can spot deceptive advertising or extravagant claims for this procedure. For example, magazine advertisements may show "successful" plug transplants by using models with minimal loss and then suggest that everyone can get the same kind of coverage.

Because we do all types of hair replacement surgery, we'll try to give you an unbiased description of this technique. We'll describe our experience with hair transplants but not try to show you all the different approaches of practitioners in the field. We'll tell you how we evaluate you for hair transplants and design your hairline, take you through a typical punch grafting pro-

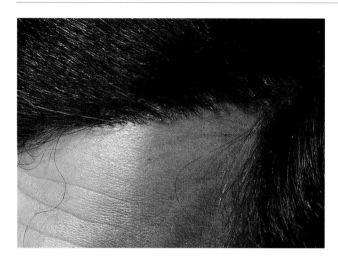
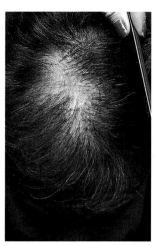

Fig. 9-1a (above left). Patient with frontal punch grafting demonstrating adequate density at the hairline.

Fig. 9-1b (above right). Parting through the transplanted scalp shows limited density immediately behind the hairline. Continued loss within the mid-scalp crown will necessitate additional work, but supply of punch grafts is diminishing.

cedure, discuss post-operative care and possible complications, and estimate how much you're likely to pay for a complete series of transplants.

How Punch Grafting Works

Punch grafting itself is straightforward. In a two-hour office procedure, 50-100 grafts about one-sixth inch in diameter are removed from the hair-bearing skin at the back of the head. Then, they are transferred to "holes" of the same size in the bald scalp—prepared by punching out and discarding small circles of skin. The grafts quickly begin connecting to blood vessels, but the hair in the grafts falls out and doesn't start to regrow for three months. The follicles will continue to produce hair because of something called donor dominance.

Basically, donor dominance means that the characteristics of your donor scalp will dominate over the characteristics of the recipient area. Thus, when hair-bearing grafts are taken from the back of your head and placed into your bald scalp, they'll continue to grow hair in their new location exactly as they would in their old, donor area. The direction of growth can be controlled simply by placing the graft into the bald scalp at the correct angle and position. Although this hair will have a different texture (usually coarser and curlier) than normal, it is otherwise quite serviceable (fig. 9-2).

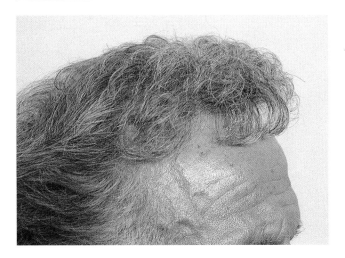

Fig. 9-2. Patient after transplants at the hairline. Note the difference in texture and curl compared to non-transplanted hair on the side of scalp.

Are Hair Transplants Right for You?

Hair transplants are not for everyone. Your doctor should thoroughly discuss punch grafting with you to make sure you have reasonable expectations. The extent of your present and future baldness (fig. 9-3), availability of donor grafts, and quality of donor hair are very important to understanding how much coverage you can expect.

Your Age — If you're a young man with little hair loss, you may want to delay transplantation until your ultimate pattern of baldness is clear. You might be tempted to begin hair replacement early because a small amount of work may temporarily eliminate baldness. But your satisfaction will be short-lived as you lose more hair later and are left with "corn rows" of sparse transplanted hair at your hairline.

The key problem with early grafting is that most of your donor hair may be used to cover thinning areas near your front hairline, leaving large areas of baldness as hair loss continues (fig. 9-4). Typically, you would have 500 to 600 small grafts available for transplantation, and up to 450 might be necessary just for the hairline and frontal scalp. Having used many of your donor grafts, you would have to fall back on scalp reductions as baldness progresses (see Chapter 8), with little likelihood of getting a satisfactory result. A better approach is to de-

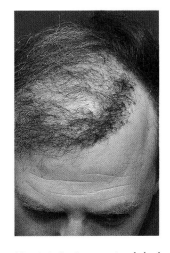

Fig. 9-3. Patient previously had punch graft transplantation to frontal scalp without anticipating his progression of male pattern baldness. We recommended additional punchgrafting.

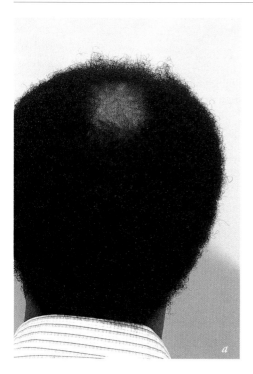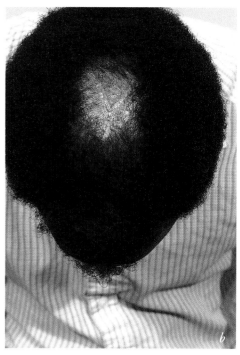

Fig. 9-4a (above left) and 9-4b (above right). Views after reduction in crown and punch grafts to treat hair loss in the frontal scalp. Only a small amount of baldness remains within the crown.

Fig. 9-4c (opposite left) and 9-4d (opposite right). Fifteen years later, male pattern baldness has extended over the entire top of the scalp. The patient's shaved head shows the size of the involved area very clearly. The progression of baldness is very critical in evaluating a patient for surgical treatment.

termine your ultimate balding pattern and then to transplant hair so it will best treat that larger eventual bald area.

Extent of Your Baldness — If you're among the rare group of people who will have only frontal (Class I) hair loss, punch grafting may give you good results. If you have or will have more than frontal loss, however, we must carefully plan the concentration and placement of your grafts to get the best coverage. First, we may want to do scalp reductions to decrease the bald area in the midscalp and crown as much as possible before transplanting. But if your scalp is not elastic enough to do much reduction, the grafts should be concentrated in your hairline and on the part side of your head. Placing the same number of grafts evenly over your scalp would leave a less dense appearance—one that probably wouldn't satisfy you. By growing your transplanted hair long and combing it across the areas of your scalp with fewer transplants, you can produce the look of light to moderate thinning—but not a full head of hair.

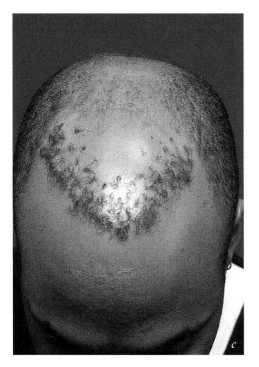
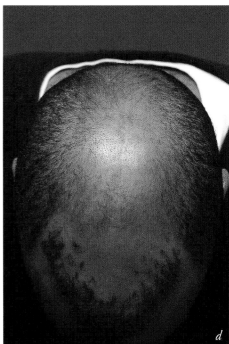

We also recommend against using "spot" grafts to fill in thinning hair. Instead, you must be willing to have your physician transplant your thinning scalp as though it were bald. The surgical shock of placing grafts may cause added hair loss and even speed up your genetically programmed pattern of baldness. Many of these lost hairs start to regrow about three months later, but they are finer and less dense (fig. 9-5). Also, the natural progression of your baldness would cause hair to fall out around the grafts, resulting in a continuing thin to balding appearance. Thus, the net gain of your single transplant operation could be insignificant.

Your Hair Quantity and Density — Obviously, for hair transplantation to work, you must have enough hair left to graft into your bald skin. Coverage depends largely on how many hairs are growing in each donor graft. On average, people have about 15 hairs per one-sixth-inch graft, but you must have at least 10 to get reasonable results. Your "safe" donor area is a conservative estimate of the hair available for healthy transplants.

Fig. 9-5 (below). Crust on punch grafts placed three weeks earlier. Hair in the punch grafts normally falls out after surgery. Surrounding hair also fell out. Hair began to grow again three months after the operation.

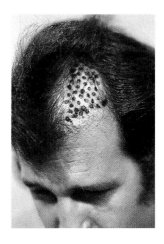

Grafts containing only your <u>fringe hair</u> (hair which is genetically programmed to fall out later) could suffer complete hair loss after transplanting, in which case they would fail in their new location and leave exposed scars behind.

Normally, the thickest hair at the middle-back part of your head would contribute grafts to cover your hairline, the center of your crown, and the part side of your scalp. Thinner hair — from the lower margins at the sides and back of your head — can go to areas where density isn't so critical and to refine the front row of your hairline. Closer to your temples, fewer grafts are taken so the skin under this sparser hair doesn't become exposed.

Evaluating density is vital for curly or kinky hair, which often looks thicker than it is. For example, the very kinky hair typical of black patients may be sparse, having only eight or nine hairs per graft. The hair shafts and follicles also curve under the outer layer of the skin, making it extremely hard to avoid injuring these underlying follicles when harvesting the grafts. For these reasons, if you have very kinky hair, you'll want to select a doctor with extensive experience in transplantation. Of course, the best approach here would be hair flaps (see Chapter 10), which are less likely to injure the underlying hair follicles.

Density in your donor area also determines whether you should have scalp reductions before or after punch grafting. If you're a borderline candidate for transplantation, with low hair density, we must be especially careful about doing scalp reductions before transferring the grafts. Reductions stretch the donor area and therefore make the donor hair less dense. In this case, we may begin punch grafting at your new hairline—which needs the most density—before reducing your scalp. On the other hand, if you have dense hair, even more transplants are available after a reduction, because this procedure stretches your donor skin while retaining enough density in the individual grafts.

Your Hair Quality — Hair quality is as important as quantity to the grafting procedure. The caliber and curl of your hair will vary over different parts of your donor area. In grafting your hairline, thin caliber hair should be used because it decreases the appearance of tufting ("rows of corn" appearance). The thicker appearance of larger caliber hair is sacrificed to avoid its much more serious disadvantage of heavy tufting. As mentioned earlier, curly or wavy hair gives the illusion of more body and greater density when this may not be the case. The coarseness of your hair is important because coarse hair covers better than fine hair.

Your Hair Color — Another key concern when deciding whether to transplant hair is your hair color. Dark hair covers better than light hair, but the tufting or "corn-row" appearance that always comes with transplanting is more apparent because of its contrast with the underlying skin. If you're a blond or redhead, your punch grafted hair may not appear as thick, but with tufting less obvious, it may look more natural. The best hair color is gray or "salt and pepper," because the density is often as high as when the hair was dark, and the now lighter color contrasts very little with the scalp.

Designing Your Hairline, Part, and Crown

A proper hairline is vital to a successful hair-replacement operation. For example, you may want a lower hairline but show little concern for your crown. Or you may not object to a slightly higher hairline, as long as you can place transplants in the entire bald area, including the crown. While taking your wishes into account, your surgeon will want to create a natural and aesthetically pleasing design.

Leonardo da Vinci divided the front view of the face into thirds. The bottom third extends from the lower border of your chin to the bottom of your nose; the middle third continues to your glabella (between the eyebrows); and the upper third continues from the glabella to your front hairline (fig. 9-6). Thus, our first rule

Fig. 9-6 (right). Facial proportion according to Leonardo da Vinci. Normal frontal hairline location is at the top limit of upper third of face. Hairline should be placed at or above this point, but not below.

Fig. 9-7a (bottom left). Patient with frontal baldness. Markings show placement of hairline with well defined, normal recession.

Fig. 9-7b (bottom right). View with head down showing gentle convex curve and location of hairline.

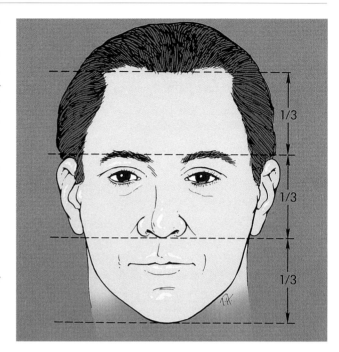

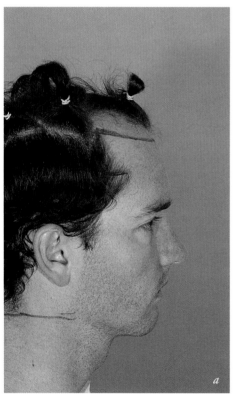

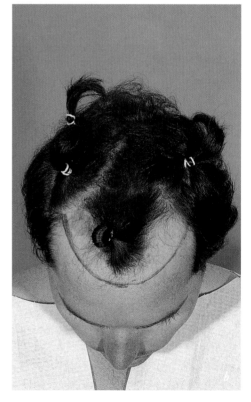

is: never place the hairline below the top border of this upper third of your face. For average adult men with no hair loss, this border would be about two and one half to two and three quarters inches above the glabella.

With few exceptions, a man's normal hairline should be a gentle convex curve (fig. 9-7). Also, your front hairline should form an acute angle where it meets the hair at your temples, making a "temporal gulf." In other words, your hairline should slant slightly downward from back to front—never upward. Blunting or rounding of this temporal gulf creates an ape-like appearance that is abnormal and almost impossible to conceal (fig. 9-8).

The curve of your hairline should be gentle—never excessive or flat. Though we've had a few patients who preferred slightly flatter hairlines, we're careful to keep them in the normal range.

Because you'll see yourself from the front view, a small difference in placement of the front hairline can alter your "look" considerably. For this reason, most surgeons draw in two or more hairlines and ask you to choose which one looks best to you—tempered, of course, by the surgeon's own judgment about the aesthetic result.

Usually, though, the hairline is placed as high as possible because this position reduces the number of punch grafts needed to cover the baldness behind it. It's better to place the hairline higher to avoid an irreversible problem. It can always be lowered with more punch grafting if your ultimate balding pattern is less than anticipated. Punch grafting can bring your hairline forward one row at a time.

Placing your hairline demands special care when scalp reductions accompany a transplant procedure. To plan for a midline reduction after grafting the hairline, the grafts are placed lower on both sides of your scalp. Reductions behind frontal grafts will elevate the junction between your hairline and temples. Thus, most doctors would rather do the reductions first, so they

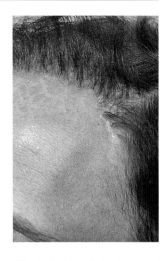

Fig. 9-8 (above). Patient had previous punch grafts with rounding of the hairline and poor hairline design. This creates an ape-like appearance.

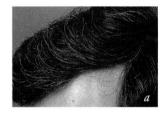

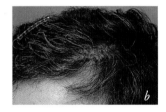

Fig. 9-9a (top). Patient with frontal transplants. Part line goes through non-transplanted hair on side of scalp.

Fig. 9-9b (above). Transplanted hair pulled aside. A part through this transplanted hair would reveal tufting.

Fig. 9-10. Four sessions are necessary to fill any area. The width of one graft separates transplants at each session.

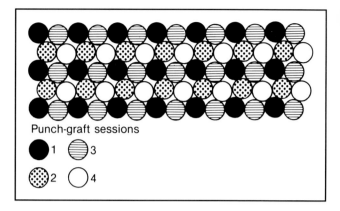

don't have to worry about later changing the contour or configuration of the hairline.

Where you part your hair is also important to transplantation. Usually, your partline would start at a point lying directly above the junction between the side and middle thirds of your eyebrow. But with transplants, you must avoid parting through the punch grafts to keep from emphasizing their tufting. If possible, you should place your part within the naturally growing, non-transplanted hair on the side of your head (fig. 9-9). Therefore, the new punch-grafted hairline and the temporal gulf should always be placed above the partline.

A bald crown is the last special concern in planning how to cover the scalp with transplants. First, because the crown contains the most elastic part of your scalp, we typically do reductions in this area before transplanting hair into it. Then, to keep the natural pattern of hair growth, we "spiral" the grafts around the crown. Again, to help "camouflage" large areas of baldness, the grafts can be concentrated on the part side of your head.

Transplanting Your Hair

Surgeons develop their own approaches to transplantation, but most will be similar to the one we describe here. You'll need at least four transplant sessions to cover any one area of baldness, with each session transferring 50 to 100 small, round grafts. For areas needing the most density, such as the hairline and partline, six or more procedures may be necessary. These transplants typically take the pattern shown in figure 9-10. As you can see, we keep some space between the grafts and offset them. Placing the grafts too close together in one session would limit blood supply to each graft, so some of the grafts wouldn't take. This sequential method of punch grafting allows adequate blood supply to keep the grafts healthy.

Although it's possible to do procedures six weeks apart, in our practice we prefer to wait three to four months between sessions, so circulation will come back to your recipient area and no grafts will be injured by the next operation. More frequent sessions will probably reduce the yield of hairs per graft and overall density.

Preparing for Transplant Surgery — To prepare for surgery, you would follow instructions similar to those in Appendix A. Before beginning the procedure, we numb your scalp with a local anesthetic. (Some physicians administer valium or an inhalant, such as "laughing gas," to calm their patients before injecting the scalp with a local anesthetic.) As in scalp reductions, we use the Derma Jet to painlessly prepare your scalp for injections of anesthetic. Other surgeons may use a Freon or Fluro-ethyl spray to "freeze" your scalp before doing these injections.

Preparing the Bald Scalp for Grafts — Once your scalp is numb, the recipient site is prepared by making incisions in your bald scalp, leaving the skin in place until it's time to harvest your donor hair. In most cases, the recipient holes are made a bit smaller than the donor grafts. These recipient holes usually expand slightly to match the size of the grafts and therefore result in a neater fit, less scar tissue, and a better cosmetic effect.

Harvesting Donor Grafts — We then remove grafts from your donor area for transplanting into the recipient sites. With efficient "harvesting" of your donor area, you should have at least 500 to 600 of these one-sixth-inch "plugs" to donate. We prefer a method of removing these grafts which produces the largest number of surviving hairs (less hair is permanently lost during surgery). The grafts are actually cut by hand, not by using a punch. We take a strip of skin from the donor hair-bearing scalp, section it into rectangular grafts, and then remove the superficial layers of skin from these grafts so they conform to the shape of the previously made holes in the recipient scalp. Small remaining sections lend themselves to micrografts or minigrafts, which we discuss later in this chapter.

You may find that some doctors allow donor sites to heal on their own. Within one to three weeks temporary crusts fall off, and the small holes left by the vacated grafts start shrinking. After a few months, the holes have formed thin, flat scars that are barely noticeable. In our practice, however, we always suture the donor area to decrease discomfort, reduce scab formation, and promote more rapid healing. Therefore no holes are left in the scalp.

All that remains after harvesting the donor grafts is to place them into the recipient sites. This is where the skill of an experienced surgeon pays off. To achieve a natural appearance and avoid tufting, the doctor must place the hair shafts at an angle of 30° to 40° relative to the surface of your scalp. The closer this angle is to 90° (perpendicular to your scalp), the worse your "cornrow" appearance becomes. At the correct angle, hair growth parallels the skin's surface, so tufting is less obvious (fig. 9-11).

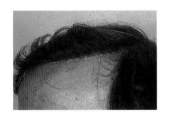

Fig. 9-11. Hairline grafts are placed at an angle of 30° to 40° relative to the plane of the scalp to reduce tufting.

Hairline grafts are even more crucial because they are the most noticeable. To get a natural-looking hairline with transplants, the direction and angle of the grafts are carefully controlled. For example, grafts at the sides of the hairline must point somewhat forward and toward the middle of your scalp. Grafts at the center of your hairline must point forward because that's the natural direction of growth. The grafts are placed smooth and flat with respect to your surrounding scalp. The surgeon must have an artistic sense and compulsive attention to detail to achieve an excellent result.

Care After Surgery

A pressure dressing is placed over the entire area when the procedure is complete. This dressing keeps your donor grafts in place and eliminates bleeding. Most patients feel little or no pain after a hair transplant operation. If you feel pressure or aching in the donor area, you can take pain medication to help relieve it. You also take medication to relieve swelling over the forehead and eyes, which may occur with transplants into your frontal scalp. Keeping your head elevated will also decrease swelling, which further reduces your discomfort.

You'll have your dressing removed the day after your surgery but will need to keep your head elevated for another day and avoid strenuous activities for another week. You should wash your hair daily, obviously being gentle in the recipient area so you don't dislodge any grafts. Frequent shampooing keeps scabbing and crusting to a minimum. If you wear a hairpiece, you may start using it again on the day after surgery as long as you don't clip it to the recipient area.

You will return to your doctor's office in one week to have all sutures removed. Crusts that form on the grafts usually fall off in two to three weeks. Any that don't fall off are easy to remove. As we mentioned earlier, the hair in your grafts will fall out in about six weeks because of the shock of surgery (fig. 9-5). New hair growth begins about three months after surgery and continues at a rate of about a half inch per month. Therefore, you'll have to wait 9-12 months after surgery to see the results of the first transplant operation. Your future transplant sessions will be done every three to four months.

You can expect a decrease in sensation and occasional numbness in your scalp immediately after surgery. Normal sensation usually returns in four to six months, but a few patients have waited up to two years for it to return completely. Rarely, a person may have some permanent loss of sensation in the scalp.

Potential Concerns

Most serious complications in punch grafting arise from poor planning and technique. For example, if your hairline is too low or is blunted and rounded at the temples, you'll need to go through some kind of "revision" surgery. Scalp reduction, forehead lifting (Chapter 11), or removing and repositioning the grafts will improve your appearance. Unfortunately, such revisions seldom are ideal.

Placing grafts at incorrect angles or in the wrong direction is another problem that can make effective styling of your hair almost impossible. When patients are referred to us for reconstructive work, we can re-cut and reposition these grafts. But reharvesting often leads to decreased yield per graft and, therefore, to a sparser appearance.

If you have inadequate circulation in your recipient area, such as a section of scarring, your transplanted hair may grow poorly. In this case, we would go more slowly with subsequent transplants, doing fewer grafts at each sitting. In many cases, though, lack of hair comes from taking too many grafts in one procedure or from poor surgical technique. Your best bet when dealing with scarred tissue is a scalp reduction or flap surgery. Flaps replace your bald area with hair-bearing scalp having improved circulation (see Chapter 10), so they are much better than transplants as a solution for this problem.

Under certain conditions, you may experience "cobblestoning," or persistent rising of the grafts above the skin, in your recipient scalp. However, this can be avoided. Cobblestoning usually occurs because your donor scalp is thicker than your recipient skin. In this case, we can thicken the recipient scalp by injecting it with saline or we can deepen the recipient holes before placing the grafts. Bleeding may also cause cobblestoning by pushing a graft above the skin, but we can easily place a suture in the surface layer of the scalp (epidermis) to keep it in position. "Cobblestoning" can be improved after surgery by "dermabrading" (shaving) the elevated graft skin.

Of course, some complications occur even in the hands of an experienced surgeon using perfect technique. For example, bleeding during surgery can be troublesome, but gentle pressure usually stops it. Sutures or treated gauze will solve any persistent bleeding, which is very rare. Although there are a few reported cases of infection following hair transplantation, the excellent blood supply in your scalp would make this very unusual. We occasionally see inflammation in a single graft—easily treated with local care. Pinkness around the edges of the grafts may last two to three months, but the final white scar is inconspicuous on all but the darkest complexions. The skin of the transplants will be a different color because they have never been tanned.

Using Minigrafts and Micrografts

Micrografts, which contain one to two individual hairs, are one of the significant advances in hair-replacement surgery over the last ten years (fig. 9-12). Although the Japanese described micrografting more than 50 years ago, the first American descriptions of it appeared in 1980. Minigrafting (small grafts with three to six hairs) is really an old technique with a new name.

Minigrafts usually fill in small areas of baldness be-

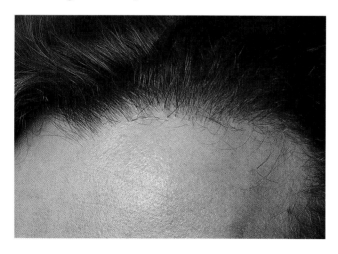

Fig. 9-12. Patient with full head of hair who had micrografts placed at hairline.

tween standard-size grafts or are used to reconstruct eyebrows or mustaches (see Chapter 14). Tufting and changes in texture aren't as obvious with these small grafts, so they provide a more natural appearance than large round grafts used alone. Also, if you have extensive baldness and simply wish to have some hair, minigrafts can be positioned randomly over your scalp—with an extra concentration in the front. In this case, we don't try to eliminate baldness; we simply give you some hair in a large bald area.

The surgical technique for minigrafts is fairly simple. After the usual preparations, we harvest a single strip of skin and then cut it into the small mini-grafts, each containing three to six hairs. We make small recipient holes by removing skin and then place the grafts. This technique reduces scarring and improves the yield of growing hairs. In fact, hair often continues to grow in micro- and minigrafts immediately after surgery. If it does fall out temporarily, it will start growing again three months later, just as in standard-size grafts.

Micrografts (one to two hairs) are most often used to refine, or "feather," the hairline after punch grafting (fig. 9-13). Micrografts employ finer, smaller-caliber donor hairs to soften the "rows of corn" appearance within the first row of standard-size grafts. They are also used to camouflage hairline scars, eyelashes, eyebrows, and mustaches.

Many doctors harvest their micrografts by punching out a standard-sized graft and then splitting the graft into smaller pieces of skin which contain one or two hairs. But we feel we can do this procedure faster by removing a single, two-millimeter-wide strip of hair-bearing skin and then cutting from it grafts containing the one or two hairs. After harvesting the micrografts, we put small holes one to two millimeters apart in the recipient scalp and use a jeweler's forceps to position them.

Some doctors report that they can place up to 900 of these micrografts in a single sitting, often using them

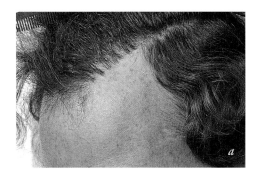 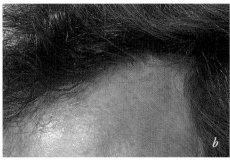

over a large bald area to give the appearance of some hair with very low density (fig. 9-14). When doctors use micrografts to soften your hairline after transplantation, they place the grafts in an irregular pattern within two or three millimeters of your previously transplanted hair. This produces the "feathering" effect typical of a naturally growing hairline. We can also use micrografts to soften the hairline after hair flap surgery, as described in Chapter 10.

Fig. 9-13a (above left). After initial sessions of punch grafts, the tufting and lack of density are very apparent.

Fig. 9-13b (above right). Mini and micrografts were subsequently used to soften the "row of corn" appearance and refine the hairline.

Incisional Slit Grafting

Recently, a procedure called incisional slit grafting has evolved. In this technique smaller grafts are used routinely to cover large areas of baldness. The grafting sessions provide a light to moderately thinning appearance—depending on your hair caliber and texture. For each session, we split full-sized round grafts into halves and quarters or harvest strips of skin and divide them into smaller grafts. These minigrafts are then placed into recipient sites. We make recipient holes in the bald scalp with a small knife and place the grafts in these incisions without removing any bald skin.

Slit grafting has some advantages over punch grafting. Because no plugs are removed from the recipient scalp, blood vessels remain intact over the entire bald area, with some observed improvement in transplant hair growth. Smaller incisions also produce smaller, usually unnoticeable, scars. With heavy use of minigrafts toward the front of the head, as well as up to

Fig. 9-14. Micrografts placed within large bald area to provide "some hair" without significantly decreasing the baldness.

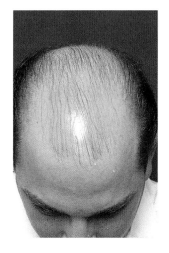

a more feathered, irregular hairline—much like that of naturally growing hair. Although this procedure can never give you the full head of hair of your youth, it can produce a more natural thinning look than traditional transplantation.

Styling and Managing Your Transplanted Hair

Most people who undergo hair transplants find they can improve the results with certain hairstyling techniques, especially for the part and hairline. You must part your hair where its growth is most dense and uniform, so parting through the transplants is unwise. A common approach is to part the hair one-half to one inch below the transplanted area and then comb the extra hair over it to create a denser appearance.

Combing near the hairline can also improve or detract from a natural look. For example, combing your hair forward in a "Caesar" style can help to disguise an unsatisfactory hairline and cover thinning areas closer to the front of your head with the thicker hair that usually grows near the back. You can also create a thickening effect without a part simply by sweeping the naturally growing hair at your temples up and gradually forward. Of course, we would recommend getting your hairline improved with additional transplants whenever possible, rather than using the temporary solution of styling.

When your transplanted hair takes on a kinky texture, it's better to "go with the flow" than to try to comb it down and keep it in place. That is, you can keep the transplanted hair fairly short and frizz it up after washing by just running your fingers through it, or even having your stylist do some permanent waving or curling to match its growth pattern.

Two other methods are available to increase the apparent fullness of your transplanted hair. You should shampoo often enough to remove oils which flatten and separate your hair. Your best bet is probably a mild conditioning shampoo because the conditioners add bulk, softness, and manageability. If your hair growth is too sparse for shampooing alone to give it a full look, you can improve your appearance by trying one of the colored sprays for tinting your scalp. These sprays dissolve in water and come in various tints to match your hair color. To use it, you part your hair to the sides in regular rows, hold the spray can about a foot away from your head, and apply the coloring in light, brief movements along the rows. The coloring reduces reflection of light from your scalp and keeps the transplanted hair from standing out against a pale, shiny background.

Paying for Transplants

As with all medical procedures, the cost of your transplants will reflect the physician's experience and active participation in your surgery, as well as the follow-up services and training of assistants. Of course, you shouldn't automatically assume the highest-priced service is also the best. Rather, base your choice on careful evaluation of the doctor, his staff, and his actual results. See live patients who originally had your type of hair and degree of baldness after their hair replacement surgery.

Variations in experience and services result in fees between $15 and $150 per graft—the customary way of charging for a transplant operation. Thus, if your complete transplant requires between 250 and 550 grafts (a typical range), your cost could run from $3,800 to as much as $80,000. Because transplants are spread over several months to several years, you can budget "as you go" payments to some extent.

A Few Last Words

Punch grafting is a relatively simple, widely practiced technique for replacing some hair in bald scalps. Once your hair is transplanted from a good donor area, this "new" hair will grow as long as your donor hair continues to grow. Because of its simplicity and availability, punch grafting may well be a good choice for you.

We've pointed out, however, that transplantation is time-consuming and unable to give you back anything close to a full head of hair, especially if your baldness is extensive. It produces hair with altered texture and could give you a "rows of corn" appearance because of tufting. Although new techniques using minigrafts and micrografts have improved the naturalness of transplants, patients often find their results unsatisfactory. For these reasons, you may decide that hair flaps — described in the next chapter — are a better, faster surgical approach to eliminating your baldness.

10.
Flap Surgery

Hair flaps are the most advanced method of hair replacement today. The pedicle flap discussed below has a dramatic cosmetic effect. Unlike transplanted hair in punch grafts, which becomes coarse and creates a tufted or "doll's-hair" appearance, flap hair continues to grow normally immediately after surgery. It has your own natural density and uniformity (no rows of corn) and doesn't fall out temporarily after surgery. Thus, a hair-flap patient has "instantaneous," luxuriant hair to replace his baldness.

A hair "flap" is simply a thin, banana-shaped strip of hair-bearing scalp — slightly more than one and a half inches wide and five to eight inches long — that is moved from the side of your head and repositioned to replace bald areas in the front, middle, or crown areas of your scalp. One end of the pedicle flap remains attached to the scalp immediately above the ear. It is rotated into position and placed in the recipient area after removal of the appropriate amount of bald skin. The area where the flap was taken is sutured together and the remaining thin scar is easily covered by growing hair (fig. 10-1).

The publication of Dr. Raymond Passot's research in 1931 marks the true beginning of flap surgery as a premier technique for hair replacement. To solve crown baldness, Passot based a short flap of hair near the back of the head and extended it forward along the side

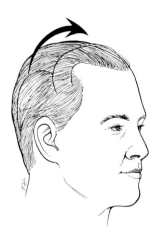

Fig. 10-1. The Fleming/Mayer Flap has been taken from the side and back of the head and then rotated to establish a new hairline after removal of bald frontal scalp skin. Surrounding hair hides the thin scar on the side of the head which remains after removal of the flap.

toward the temple. He kept the flap rooted in a pedicle, or pivot of skin, at the back and then swung it up and across the crown—placing it into a like opening which he had created on the bald scalp. Several weeks later, he did a second flap from the opposite side and brought it up to meet the other flap at the midline of the patient's head. Because of the scalp's elasticity, he was able to pull together the edges of the skin from which each flap was lifted and simply suture it closed.

To correct frontal baldness, Passot used flaps based near the temples and extending along the sides of the head. In this case, he kept the flaps rooted at the front and swung them up and forward to meet across the frontal scalp, creating a new hairline. As we'll describe in more detail later, he provided these flaps with their own blood supply by basing them on the artery near the surface of your skin which begins at the temples and continues back along the sides of your head.

The next important development in flap surgery came in 1957, when Dr. E. S. Lamont described using flaps similar to Passot's, but only after "delaying" them twice before rotating them into their new position across the front hairline. A "delay" is the procedure by which a surgeon makes incisions around the edges of a piece of tissue, so the tissue is isolated from surrounding skin except at the point of attachment at its base. Blood flow then increases through this point of attachment and continues after the flap is rotated, thus improving the ultimate health of the flap. As you'll see in the section on delays below, this has become a standard part of our technique in using longer flaps for hair replacement.

In 1975, a South American doctor named Jose Juri presented his work with long flaps, which extended from near the temples to the back of the head and included the artery mentioned above. His flaps were slightly more than an inch and a half wide and were also twice delayed. Juri's methods produced outstanding results with only minor complications, so we and others began working with this concept in the United States.

As we studied the Juri flap, we recognized that we could improve it. Since the late 1970s, we've continued to modify Juri's original design to produce superior results.

Surgical Procedure for the Fleming/Mayer Flap

Flap Delays — As mentioned earlier, we always do two delays before rotating a Fleming/Mayer Flap into its new position on the bald scalp. After each delay, blood flow concentrates and increases along the length of the flap. Once it's rotated, the flap continues to be nourished by this strong supply of blood and therefore survives well in its new location.

If we don't delay the flap twice we risk damage to it, as well as permanent hair loss. In thousands of flap procedures for patients who haven't had previous surgery, only two permanently lost any hair. One was a three-pack-a-day smoker with impaired circulation. We do delays from six to eight days apart. One week after the second delay, we rotate the flap.

Procedure for First Delay — First, we design your new hairline. Then, we choose the side from which to take your flap and draw it on your scalp, using the proper curvature and length to achieve the hairline we've designed. The flap is based on the superficial temporal artery that extends from the temple. We keep the flap well within the donor area, taking into consideration possible future hair loss as your baldness progresses (fig. 10-2).

Most patients need only local anesthesia—as previously described for other procedures—to go through the first and second delay. The entire procedure takes one and a half hours, but this includes designing the hairline and the flap. The actual surgery takes only about 30 minutes. We do the incisions parallel to your hair follicles to avoid hair damage and keep scars narrow. In addition, we bevel these incisions, so hair will grow through the scars and cover them. Finally, we scratch the outline of the flap tail in the skin, making it

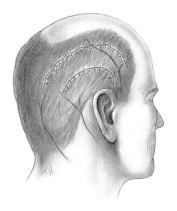

Fig. 10-2. First delay of Fleming/Mayer Flap. The superficial temporal artery is within the center of the flap at its base. Approximately three-fourths of the flap has been incised. We use an irregular incision along the top border because it will correspond to the irregular design of the new hairline.

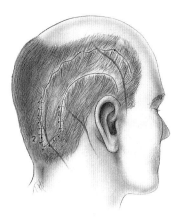

Fig. 10-3. Second delay of Fleming/Mayer Flap. The back 25-30 percent of the flap is incised and then immediately closed.

easy to find when we do the second delay one week later.

You wear a dressing home from this surgery, take your pain medication when necessary, and come back the next morning for removal of the dressing. You can then return to your hotel or home, gently wash your hair, and go back to work—as long as you avoid strenuous activity. Surgical clips used in the procedure won't be noticeable. Both this procedure and the second delay are undetectable within your hair.

Procedure for Second Delay — One week later, you come back to the operating room, receive the same preparation and local anesthesia, and undergo the second delay. Here, in a 30-minute procedure, we simply make incisions around the tail of the flap, leaving the other end of the flap attached above the ear. Again, this delay improves the flow of blood through the flap. We then use surgical clips to close the incisions (fig. 10-3).

Your activities and discomfort after this delay are identical to those after the first. On the morning after surgery, you return to have the dressings removed, go back to your home or hotel, wash your hair with regular shampoo, and either blow-dry (cool setting) or air-dry your hair. Again, you can return to work immediately but need to avoid exercise. You won't have any noticeable signs of having had surgery.

Rotating the Flap — One week after the second delay, or two weeks from the day we started, you return to have your flap transposed to the top of your head—a procedure that takes about two and a half hours. You have nothing to eat or drink after midnight the night before surgery but wash your hair as usual the morning of surgery. Before you go into the operating room, we draw your hairline and show it to you for approval one last time before transposing the flap.

In this procedure you receive light general anesthesia, after which we lift the flap, remove a matching amount of your bald scalp, and rotate the flap into place. Finally, we close the donor area by stretching your hair-bearing skin and the skin behind your ear to close the

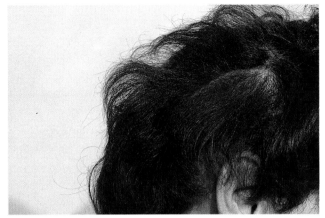

Fig. 10-4 (left). Hair combed back shows scar after the donor closure has healed. Hair will hide this incision.

Fig. 10-5a (below). Patient after removal of flap which was rotated to establish a new hairline. A small skin graft was placed in the back of the donor closure to avoid tension on the scalp. The surrounding hair hides the donor graft.

Fig. 10-5b (bottom). The small graft has been removed after the scalp regained its normal elasticity.

defect created by surgery (fig. 10-4). If the lower hairline behind your ear is elevated too much as we close the defect after flap removal, or if the closure would otherwise place too much tension on your scalp, we use a small, temporary skin graft to fill the area (fig. 10-5). Your hair easily covers this graft so it's not noticeable, and we remove it after your scalp has regained its normal elasticity—usually within three to four months.

Once we've lifted your flap and closed your donor area, we can rotate the flap and place it into the prepared area where your bald scalp was removed. We bevel the incisions along the hairline so your hair will grow from follicles buried beneath, and in front of, the skin closure. This growth establishes a new hairline that camouflages the scar (fig. 10-6). Some reaction and redness occur at the hairline incision as the hair grows through and in front of it. This is minor and temporary, lasting about six weeks (fig. 10-7).

After Surgery — Because you've had a light general anesthesia for this procedure, we keep you in the recovery room for one to two hours following surgery and then release you to a recovery center. If you prefer to go home, or to a hotel if you're from out of town, you must have a friend or family member stay with you. You'll take medication for pain, antibiotics to prevent infection, and anti-swelling medication. The next morning, and again 48 hours after surgery, you return to have

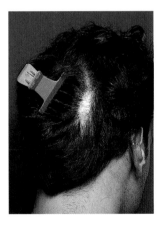

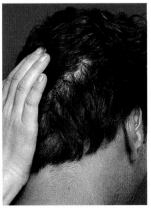

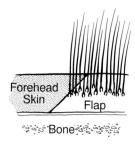

Fig. 10-6. Hairline closure. The hairline incision is beveled to bury hair follicles under the skin closure. These follicles produce hair that establishes the new hairline and camouflages the scar. Hair will grow through and in front of the hairline incision.

your dressings changed.

On the third or fourth day after surgery, you can remove this last set of dressings, wash your hair, blow-dry on the cool setting, and return to most of your normal activities. Because the hair within the flap doesn't stop growing, you will have immediate coverage and can style your hair to cover the healing hairline incision. We remove all hairline sutures on the sixth day, after which you can go to work, or back home if you live elsewhere. Ten to twelve days after surgery, all remaining surgical clips are removed by us, a friend, or a family member. Although you can begin exercising lightly after two to three weeks, we recommend against <u>heavy</u> exercise for a month.

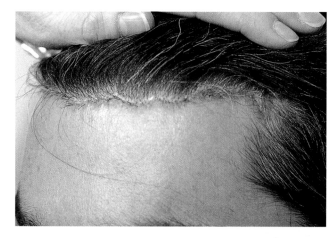

Fig. 10-7a. Hairline shortly after flap placement. Some redness is present as the hair grows through the hairline incision.

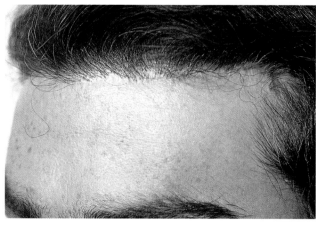

Fig. 10-7b. Hairline one month later with resolution of reaction and redness. Irregularity mimics contour of a naturally occurring hairline.

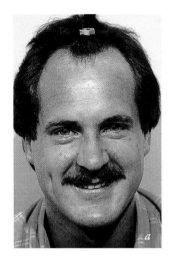

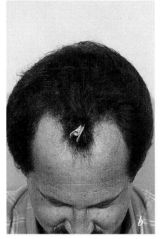

Figs. 10-8a and 10-8b. Pre-operative views of patient with frontal baldness.

Figs. 10-8c, 10-8d, and 10-8e. Patient seven years after Flap rotation. Hair parted shows normal uniform density which blends with surrounding hair. One flap eliminated the baldness.

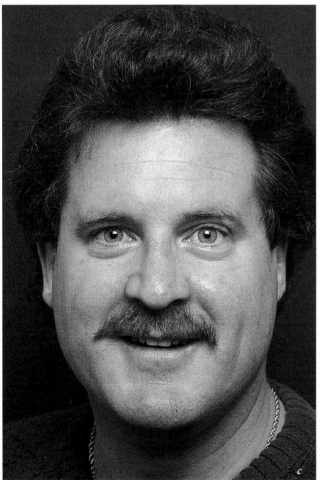

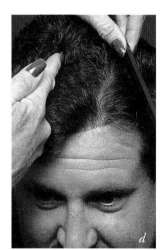

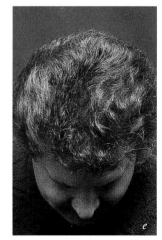

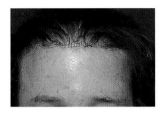

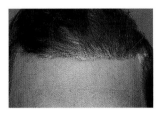

Fig. 10-9a (top). Patient six days after surgery with hair combed back immediately before removal of hairline sutures. Small bump or "dog ear" present at end of hairline. Fig. 10-9b (above). Same patient three weeks after surgery with redness along hairline and decrease in size of dog ear. The dog ear is easily concealed with the surrounding hair.

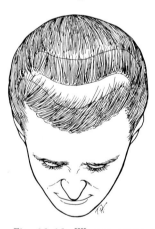

Fig. 10-10. We can rotate a second flap from the opposite side of the scalp and place it one to one and a quarter inches behind the front flap.

A few post-operative symptoms are worth noting. You may have some temporary swelling in the side of your neck behind the ear, but it's usually not noticeable to others. Although there is virtually no pain after 24 hours, you may have some tightness over this same area for several weeks.

If you have only frontal baldness, you're done. All of your bald skin is gone, and you now have natural hair growing in its place. Also, unlike what often happens with punch grafting, you'll have no further hair loss in this area for the rest of your life (fig. 10-8).

The Last Step — When the flap is rotated, a slight bulge of scalp occurs at the front edge of the flap (fig. 10-9). This occurs because the flap skin is rotated back upon itself to create the hairline. We call this small bump a "dog-ear." Immediately after surgery your hair easily covers the dog-ear. At six weeks after flap-rotation surgery, we remove it. Both the procedure to eliminate the dog-ear and to remove the donor graft are minor, so you can return to work the day after surgery.

Doing a Second Flap (Class III Baldness)

If your baldness progresses after you have your first flap, you can decide when this baldness bothers you enough to have a second flap surgery. If you're already bald over the top of your head and wish to proceed as quickly as possible, we wait three months after transposing the first flap before beginning the second (fig. 10-10). Your scalp needs this much time to regain enough elasticity for another flap procedure.

We do two delays and then transpose this flap just as we did before, but the procedure is simpler. This second flap will be about one to one and a quarter inches behind the first. It will also follow the curvature of the first flap, although we can vary it a bit to match asymmetries in the balding pattern or frontal hairline. The dog-ear for the second flap is much smaller because we don't have to rotate the flap back upon itself as we do when creating the ideal hairline. Because it is so much smaller,

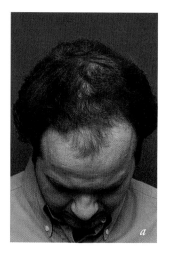
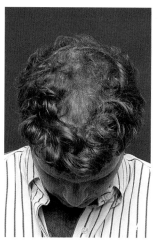

Fig. 10-11a. Pre-operative showing extensive hair loss.

Fig. 10-11b. Same patient after one Fleming/Mayer Flap. Patient has curly hair which falls over new hairline. When baldness progresses, a second flap will be done.

it resolves on its own and does not require a separate procedure.

Activities after your second flap surgery are the same as for the first except that they're less restrictive. For example, you can return to work on the third or fourth day—rather than the sixth—and you have no hairline stitches to be removed.

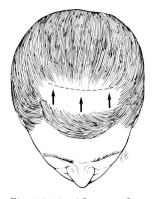

Fig. 10-12. After one flap is done and baldness progresses, a reduction behind the flap can help eliminate the balding area.

Scalp Reductions and Flap Surgery

To help eliminate balding areas between or behind flaps, we use a procedure similar in surgical technique to the reductions described in Chapter Eight. For example, suppose baldness progresses behind your frontal flap. In this case, we can remove nearly an inch of bald skin behind the flap with scalp reductions while stretching the front flap toward the back of your head. As long as you have good hair on your mid-scalp and crown, that's all you'll need at this point (figs. 10-11, 10-12). Of course, if your baldness continues to progress, a second flap would be necessary.

If you've had two flaps, we can do reductions between the flaps and remove all intervening bald scalp (fig. 10-13). Again, we would stretch the front flap back to the second flap, thus increasing its width from about one and three quarters inches to more than two inches. We can do the first of these reductions six to 12 weeks

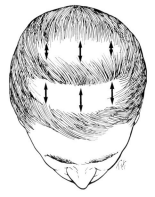

Fig. 10-13. Reductions between flaps and behind the second flap can eliminate the entire area of baldness in most patients.

Fig. 10-14a. Pre-operative view.

Fig. 10-14b. After scalp reduction surgery, the size of the donor area has been increased while simultaneously decreasing the area of scalp involved with male pattern baldness.

Fig. 10-14c. After one Fleming/Mayer Flap.

Fig. 10-14d. After two Fleming/Mayer Flaps.

Fig. 10-4e. Scalp reductions have been performed eliminating the alopecia.

Fig. 10-14f. Hair parted showing normal uniform thickness over scalp.

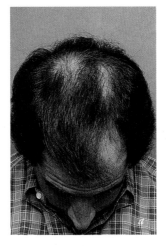
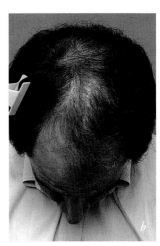
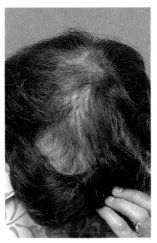
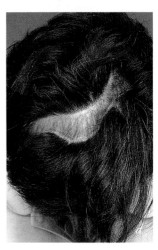
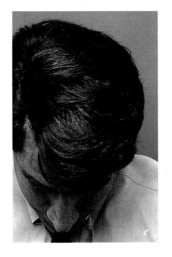
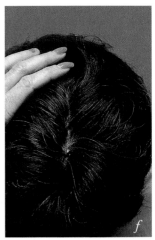

after we rotate your second flap. Then, we wait three months before doing another one, so your scalp can regain its elasticity.

Another option is to reduce bald skin behind your second flap. This reduction can take place three months after rotation of the flap. Usually, though, patients want to start reducing baldness between flaps first, because hair from the second flap adequately covers the crown. By stretching the second flap and the surrounding scalp into the crown area, we can totally remove all your Class III baldness (fig. 10-14), unless you have a very large bald area. In that case, we eliminate all of your bald area except residual baldness in your crown. It's important to note, however, that even before reduction between the flaps, you can easily style your hair so it looks full and very natural, covering all of the remaining bald scalp.

Designing the Fleming/Mayer Flap

Although all flaps follow the general description at the beginning of this chapter, certain conditions may alter our design of flaps and related procedures to cover your bald scalp.

Your Age and Ultimate Balding Pattern — As we pointed out in Chapter Three, if you're young (mid-20s) and haven't established your ultimate balding pattern, it's best to wait until we can determine what part of your hair will remain. We are always conservative in drawing a flap in your donor area so we don't include "fringe hair"—thinner hair at the border between bald scalp and normally growing hair on the sides and back of your head. This fringe may fall out later and damage the cosmetic effect of the flap and scalp.

Height of Your Donor Area and Width of Crown Baldness — We would like a height of at least four inches of good hair from which to take one and a half to one and three quarters inches of flap. If you have thin, poor-density hair that is less than four inches high, you may not be a candidate for Fleming/Mayer Flap surgery, although you may be eligible for "short flaps" un-

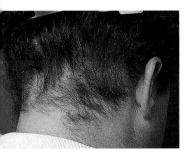

Fig. 10-15. Patient with very low density hair below and behind the ear. Design would avoid this area.

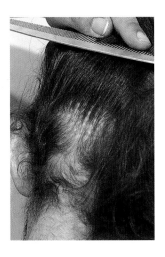

Fig. 10-16. Patient has circular scars within the donor scalp from previous harvesting of punch grafts. If possible, we avoid these scars when designing the Fleming/Mayer Flap. In many cases tissue expansion will minimize the use of scarred donor scalp (see Chapter 12).

der certain circumstances (Chapter 13). But if you have dense hair that is between three and four inches high, we can use reductions or tissue expansion before surgery to increase your donor area and still keep enough density for the flaps.

Size of Your Head and Length of Your Front Hairline — These two dimensions combine to determine how we can design your hair flap. You may have a large head with a long expanse between your temples; if so, you'll need a longer flap to establish a new hairline and, therefore, a larger donor area. As noted in Chapters 8 and 12, we can use tissue expansion and scalp reductions before developing your flap to compensate for this larger bald area.

Location of Your Temporal Artery — More than 95 percent of our patients have a temporal artery that curves up over the ear and then downward toward the back of the head. If you were among the five percent of people whose artery differs from this pattern, we would alter our design to keep it within the flap.

Quality of Hair Behind Your Ears and Near Your Neck — Our flap design varies to make sure we include hair of the highest quality. In other words, we can move the flap higher or lower on the side of your head to keep the thickest, densest hair within it (fig. 10-15).

Elasticity of Your Scalp — As we've said, the more elastic your scalp the more bald skin we can remove with reductions before doing the flap procedure. Thus, your flap would need to eliminate less remaining baldness, which in turn gives us more flexibility in designing its size and shape.

Scars or Prior Hair-Replacement Procedures — Because scars reduce circulation in the scalp, they limit where we can design the flap. Scars will always exist after punch grafting or flap surgery (fig. 10-16), so if you've had these procedures done, we try to avoid the scarred areas. If we can't avoid them completely, we want to keep the scarring to a minimum within the flap. In some cases, however, we may need to accept some scarring at the end of the flap. In these cases, tissue expansion before flap surgery can produce enough "new scalp" (see Chapter 12).

Your Wishes — We want to work with you to establish a hairline that meets your needs and is within the bounds of good aesthetic taste, so we discuss this issue carefully with you during flap design. To obtain the best possible appearance, we follow established principles of hairline design and placement. Proper height of the hairline, its position in relation to your partline, the correct angle where it meets the temples, and a gentle curve across your forehead all contribute to an artistic, pleasing outcome.

Micrografts and Flap Surgery

Our development of the irregular hairline has reduced the problem of "abruptness" in flap surgery—a sharp division between bare scalp and thick hair growing from the flap. We get excellent results even in patients with very thick hair. Still, one or two percent of our patients want an even softer hairline than we can give them with our flap procedure. For these patients, we do two or three sessions of micrografts (grafts with one or two hairs) along the front edge of the flap to soften or "feather" the edge (fig. 10-17).

The results here are superior to those we can achieve with punch-graft surgery. These micrografts are in front of an already irregular hairline and thick, full hair which has no "rows of corn" look or change to a coarse texture. That's why, even without micrografts, most of our pa-

Fig. 10-17a (bottom left) and Fig. 10-17b (bottom right). The irregular design of the flap has already softened the abruptness at the newly established flap hairline. In some patients we do micrografts to further soften or feather the hairline, as seen in the hairlines of these two patients.

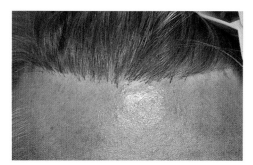
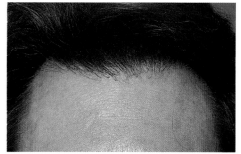

FLAP SURGERY Q & A

Q: What about skin damage?

A: Because this flap maintains blood flow through a self-contained artery, it's extremely rare to have skin damage (necrosis). Usually, when we've seen this problem in patients referred to us by other doctors, it's come from taking a flap without the temporal artery or from making the flap too narrow. We've had only two patients—one a heavy smoker—who lost part of the end of their flaps because of necrosis (skin loss). In these cases, we used a small flap from the other side to repair the damaged section of the original flap.

Q: Will I have temporary hair loss?

A: Rarely, you may have temporary loss in a small part of the flap or in your donor area because of surgical shock. As long as there is no damage to the skin itself, your hair will begin growing back within a few weeks. Although a few people may temporarily lose hair with any scalp procedure, we can usually minimize it by being careful not to interfere with circulation when closing incisions and applying dressings.

Q: Do flap patients lose a lot of blood?

A: Hair flap patients lose very little blood compared to those undergoing other surgeries. Occasionally a patient may have a hematoma (as occurs in a facelift operation). This almost always happens in the recovery room and is treated by stopping the oozing. The flap has never been affected.

Q: Is infection a problem?

A: This is a very rare and minor problem, requiring treatment with antibiotics.

Q: Are the scars visible?

A: Careful technique in closure usually keeps scars narrow and within the hair.

Q: Will there be any numbness?

A: Yes—behind your new hairline and above the donor area, but it goes away over several months to a year. You'll experience some sensitivity as the sensation returns to these areas. Occasionally, a patient may have a small area of mild permanent loss of sensation. None of our patients has considered this a serious problem.

Q: Is smoking a problem?

A: Smoking definitely slows down circulation. As mentioned earlier, our patient who lost more than an inch off the end of his flap was a heavy smoker. If you're unwilling or unable to stop smoking two weeks before and two weeks after the surgery, we recommend against having flap surgery. Your doctor may do a flap for you anyway, but he should warn you that part of the flap might die.

Q: Are prior transplants a problem?

A: We see many people who come to us dissatisfied with previous transplants and wanting a flap. Most are able to have flap surgery but some aren't. Your candidacy will depend on an individual evaluation.

tients wear their hair combed back—instead of forward as they do with punch grafting to camouflage the tufting of the punch grafts and the lack of normal density.

Doing a Crown Flap

We can start with a flap to replace your crown baldness if you are genetically programmed to have crown baldness <u>only</u> (fig. 10-18). If we think you'll have frontal baldness later, we prefer to begin with a frontal flap because only two flaps are available (one from each side of the head). Starting at your crown and then later moving to your front hairline would create a large area of baldness between the flaps. We may do scalp reductions before the flaps.

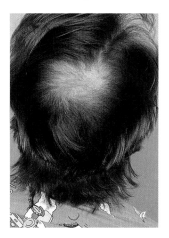
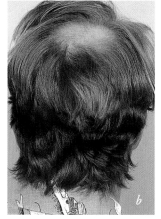
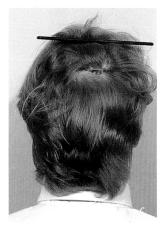
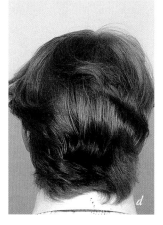

Fig. 10-18a and 10-18b. Views before flap surgery for a bald crown.

Fig. 10-18c. One week after Fleming/Mayer Flap surgery. Flap hair is elevated for critical evaluation of residual baldness. Later a scalp reduction procedure will remove the bald skin.

Fig. 10-18d. Same view, with comb removed, shows excellent cosmetic results without scalp reduction.

HAIR FLAPS VS. PUNCH GRAFTS

Long flaps have several major advantages over punch grafting, even when the latter is combined with extensive scalp reductions. Extensive scalp reductions don't give as much height in the hair over your mid-scalp and crown. In fact, they leave hair at an acute angle, so it always wants to part to the side and rear, laying flat on your head. Also, a flap gives you more height and a natural hairline with greater density and better texture. We recommend short flaps only for special applications. We feel two Fleming/Mayer Flaps combined with standard reductions remove the most bald skin and replace it with the largest possible amount of uniform, high-density, normally textured hair.

HAIR FLAPS	PUNCH GRAFTS
• Results are immediate, with no temporary hair loss. Patient returns to work four to six days after flap with dense, natural hair.	• Transplant hair falls out and takes three months to start growing. Must cover with styling or hair addition for up to two years.
• No "rows of corn".	• Corn-row "tufts."
• Can comb hair in any direction, even straight back, with natural appearance.	• Must style to cover plugs' "corn row" appearance and cover relative thinness.
• Surgery is undetectable even when hair is blown or wet.	• Plugs visible when hair is blown or parted through the transplanted hair.
• Procedure complete within a few weeks if patient has only frontal baldness.	• Usually takes two to three years to complete the entire procedure.
• No change in hair texture.	• Hair is kinky and wiry.
• Greater hair density. Thick, natural hair.	• At best, 50% density.
• Patient never requires more work in flap area.	• Continual hair loss in "plug" areas requires future procedures.
• Cost compares to or is less than equivalent number of plugs needed, with much better and more immediate results.	• Cost $15-$150 per plug but can be spread over the years needed to complete the process.

Design of a crown flap is very much like any other Fleming/Mayer Flap except that it's about an inch shorter. After doing two delays, we transpose the crown flap just as we do with a front flap. We place this flap at the front part of your crown, so your hair will grow over any remaining bald scalp behind it until we do scalp reductions, stretch the flap, and remove this baldness completely.

Dressings and removal of sutures are exactly like those for the frontal flap except there are no hairline sutures to remove. Typically, you'll return to work in three or four days without noticeable signs of having gone through flap surgery.

Styling Your Hair After Flap Surgery

Because hair in a flap keeps its thickness and uniform density, you have few limitations in styling your hair after flap surgery. You'll need to style your hair over your new hairline for several weeks until the redness along the incision disappears and the hair grows through and in front of the incision. You'll also need to comb or brush your hair over the dog-ear discussed above until we remove it six weeks later. If you have a remaining bald area behind your first flap, you'll probably want to comb the flap hair back over this bald area until you have your second flap. Some patients who have previously worn a hair addition will cut off the front part of the addition and wear the back part behind the front flap until they receive their second flap.

After this initial period, you'll be able to part your hair on the side, or even in the middle. Because hair from the flap grows in front of the incision, you can comb your hair back, exposing part or all of your hairline. With the texture of the flap hair unchanged, you'll also have no contrast between the front and side hair.

It's true that the direction of hair within a flap will be different from your original hairline. Instead of growing forward or toward the front side of your head, flap hair grows toward the back of your head in the first third of the flap and sideways and backward in the rest. But this change in direction requires no adjustment if you comb your hair back, have curly hair, or choose to have a permanent after flap surgery. If you wish to comb your hair forward and to the side, you can simply adjust your part to obtain a natural style. Because of the natural density and uniformity, styling is quite minimal especially when compared to patients with punch grafts.

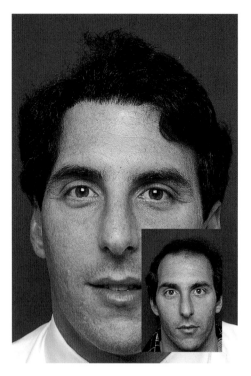

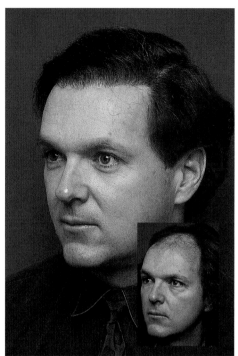

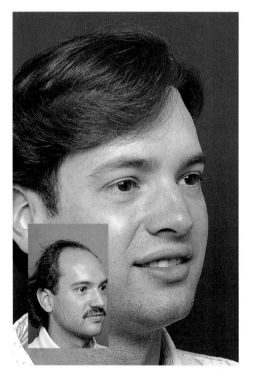

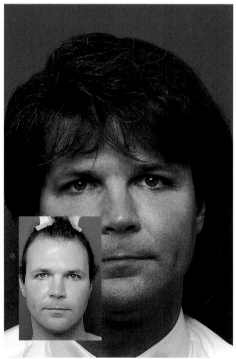

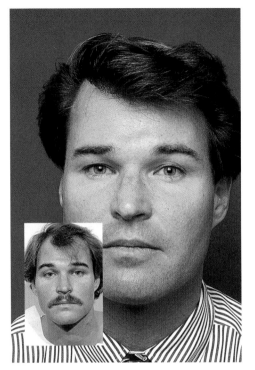

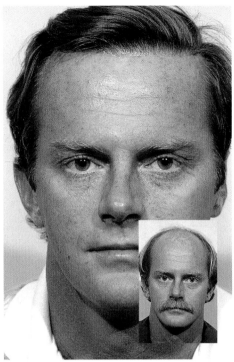

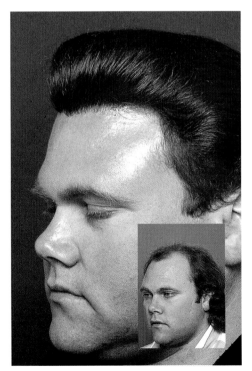

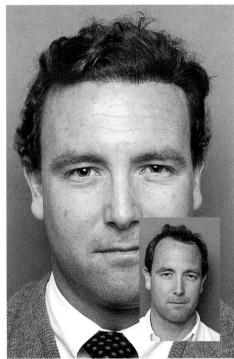

Figs. 10-19 through 10-26 (previous pages). Before and after views of patients who have undergone Fleming/Mayer Flap surgery.

A Final Word About Flaps

When we began our careers in hair-replacement surgery, we could offer people only transplantation. Scalp reductions, plus better techniques and equipment, have improved this procedure. But the disadvantages of punch grafting still make it less than completely satisfactory. Perhaps that's why each year we see more surgeons developing practices using long flaps.

Our design has enough distinctive features to have gained its own name in the medical community: the Fleming/Mayer Flap. For example, we vary the width of the flap if necessary to treat larger bald areas and we create an irregular hairline for a more natural look. To enhance appearance even more, we often do forehead or eyebrow lifts before hair-replacement surgery. We've also improved scalp-reduction patterns and employed reductions and tissue expansion before rotating a flap to achieve better results. Finally, we use skin grafts in closing the hair donor area to place less tension on incisions and promote healing.

Twenty years from now, we believe most surgery to replace hair will involve flaps, with or without tissue expansion (Chapter 12) and forehead lifting (Chapter 11). Although we do all methods of hair-replacement surgery, we believe that flaps provide the greatest advantages, the fewest disadvantages, and the most natural results for most patients with male-pattern baldness (figs. 10-19 through 10-26).

11.
The Forehead Lift

People often tell us they look sad and tired all the time. That's because the upper one-third of the face--consisting of the forehead, eyebrows, and eyelids--is the first area to show aging. The forehead develops deep creases, the eyebrows fall, and the upper eyelids become heavy and hooded. Blepharoplasty surgery (removing excess eyelid skin) improves the appearance of the eyes, but the brows remain low, and the tired look persists (fig. 11-1). On the other hand, a forehead lift places the brows in their ideal position and decreases the amount of skin in the upper eyelid with one operation. Thus, many seek correction of this problem through forehead lifting. Because this procedure combines well with hair transplantation or flap surgery to create a more youthful appearance, we'll discuss it briefly here.

This procedure has continuously improved. With our work in hair replacement surgery, we developed two operations for forehead lifting. One procedure is for women and men with a full head of hair; the other technique is for bald men. Now, we can raise or lower your front hairline while raising your eyebrows, decreasing wrinkles, and eliminating the excess skin that often makes us look tired or sad with aging. The forehead lift is now more productive than just the traditional facelift, and its results last far longer than results on the lower two-thirds of the face (fig. 11-2).

Fig. 11-1a. Patient who came to our office after having upper eyelid blepharoplasty. In addition to some excess skin of the upper eyelids, her main problem is the low position of the eyebrows which gives a heavy, tired appearance to her eyes.

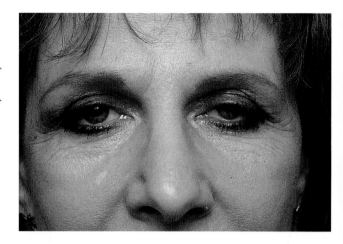

Fig. 11-1b. This photo was taken immediately after "a." She is holding her forehead and eyebrows up using fingers at her hairline. This clearly demonstrates the advantages of a forehead browlift, placing the brows in their ideal position.

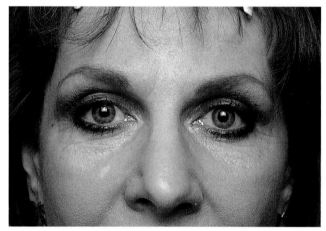

Fig. 11-2a (right). Through aging the skin loses elasticity and muscle tone. In addition to low eyebrows the patient has deep forehead grooves and frown lines. She also has facial relaxation with increased facial grooves and excess skin.

Fig. 11-2b (far right). Post-operatively patient had a forehead/eyebrow lift and facelift (cheek/necklift) surgery.

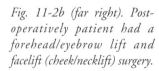
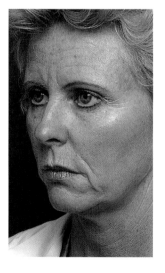
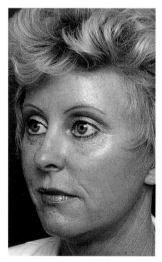

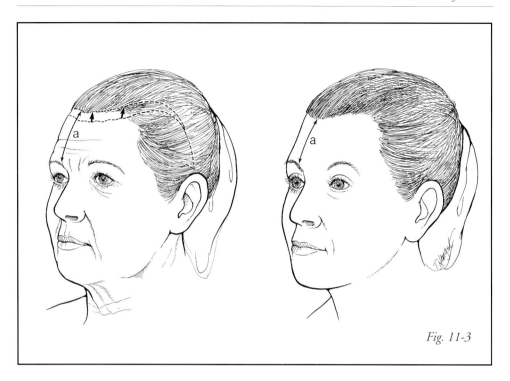

Fig. 11-3

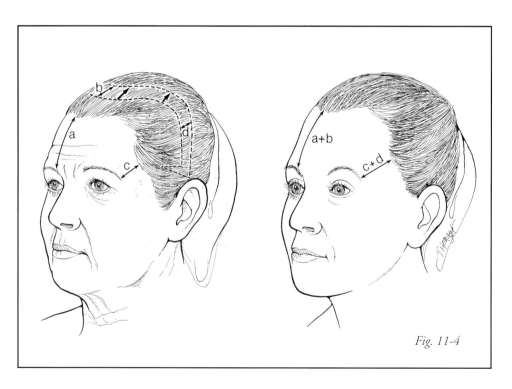

Fig. 11-4

Fig. 11-3 (previous page top). Forehead lift using the hairline incision. The hairline stays in the same position after we raise the eyebrows and remove the skin between the dotted lines. The distance "a" (the height of the forehead) is identical after surgery. Only the bald forehead skin is removed. In this way the frontal and sideburn hairlines remain in approximately the same position after lifting the forehead and eyebrows.

Fig. 11-4 (previous page bottom). Forehead lift using the older technique of incising within the hair. Good frontal hair is removed between the dotted lines to raise the eyebrows and forehead. The height of the forehead increases from "a" to "a plus b" and "c" to "c plus d" after removal of the hair-bearing skin. Therefore the frontal and sideburn hairlines are raised as a result of the operation.

Procedure for the Forehead Lift

Our surgical techniques vary somewhat for women and men, but the basic procedure for both is quite similar. Using a light general anesthesia, we create an incision at the hairline for most women having a forehead lift. We loosen the forehead skin, remove wrinkles, and do any other necessary contouring. We then lift the forehead, place the brows in the proper position, and remove excess skin (fig. 11-3).

Most women have hairlines at the proper position or too high. We developed this forehead lift and hairline incision to create the best hairline location. If the hairline is too high, we can lower it; if it is at the right level, we can maintain it at the proper position. If we want to raise or lower the hairline, it's possible to move the scalp up or down before removing excess skin, bringing the edges back together, and closing the incision. In this way we are able to retain a woman's best hair (because we're removing only the bald forehead skin), unlike other forehead lifts that remove a lot of a woman's best frontal hair (fig. 11-4).

Value of the Irregular Hairline Incision

We bevel the hairline incision so hair follicles are under the skin closure (fig. 11-5). As a result, these follicles produce hair that will grow through and in front of

Fig. 11-5a. Pre-operative patient.

Fig. 11-5b. Post-operative view after forehead lift using hairline incision. This woman is able to continue to wear her hair brushed back because the height of the forehead is unchanged and the scar is not visible, camouflaged by hair which grows through that incision.

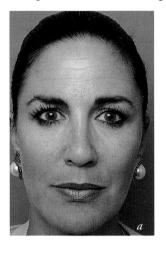
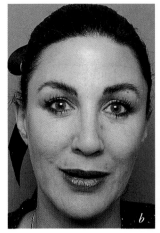

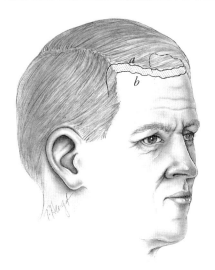

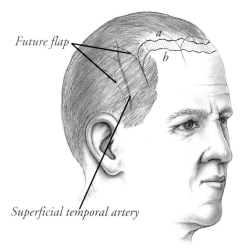

Future flap

Superficial temporal artery

the line to camouflage the incision. By using this irregular hairline incision, shown here and in Chapter 10, we leave patients with a forehead lifting scar that's hidden by their hair which grows through and in front of the scar. With a proper incision, the hair maintains exactly the same direction and quality of growth as before the procedure.

Variations for Men

We vary this incision for men depending on their needs. For example, some men have a natural hairline and will never have any baldness. In these cases, we bring the hairline incision into the hair at the temples only far enough to loosen the forehead skin, stretch it upward, and remove any excess. In this way, we remove only the bald forehead skin and maintain the natural established hairline in its normal position (fig. 11-6).

Another category of male patients consists of those who will be treated for frontal baldness with flap surgery. Many of these men choose to have a forehead lift before hair replacement surgery because this combination is convenient, cost-effective, and capable of restoring a more youthful appearance (fig. 11-8). In this case, as you can see in figure 11-7, we draw off the future flaps and make the forehead lift incisions so they end in the

Fig. 11-6 (above left). Forehead lift using the hairline incision. In a man with a full head of hair, we incise along line "a" and remove the bald forehead skin between line "a" and "b" to raise the eyebrows and forehead. The hairline position doesn't change.

Fig. 11-7 (above right). Forehead lift using hairline incision in a man with frontal baldness. Both future Fleming/Mayer Flaps are drawn with the superficial temporal artery located centrally. The incision for the hairline is along the patient's existing hairline "a" or within bald frontal scalp. We remove this scalp after transposing the Fleming/Mayer Flap. We excise bald skin between "a" and "b" while closing along line "a". Scar will be excised a few weeks later when transposing the Fleming/Mayer Flap.

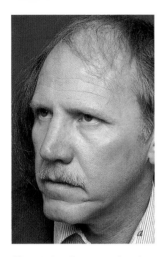

Fig. 11-8a. Pre-operative view of a patient with frontal baldness and facial aging.

Fig. 11-8b. Patient after forehead lift, rotation of Fleming/Mayer Flap to eliminate frontal baldness, and facelift surgery. Hair replacement surgery plus a forehead lift and facelift restore a more youthful appearance.

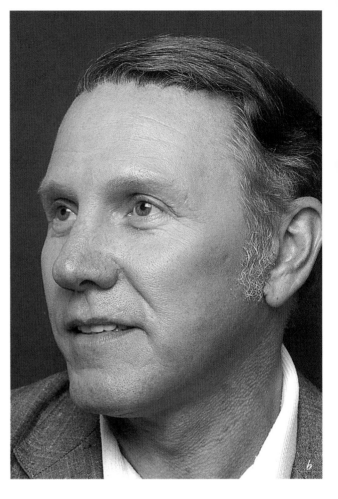

temporal hair along the upper edge of the flaps. We remove the bald skin between incision lines a and b and then close along a. About four to six weeks later, we start the flap procedure. This sequence allows removal of the scar created by the forehead lift when we rotate the flap into its final position at the hairline.

After Forehead-Lift Surgery

The forehead lift takes about one hour to complete. Your head will be wrapped in a light dressing, and you can go home with a family member under supervised care or to a separate facility for postoperative care. You'll apply ice over your eyes to control swelling for 24 hours, after which you return to the office for removal of the dressings. You will wash your hair as soon as the dressings have been removed. You will return to work in two to seven days. We remove the hairline sutures after six days and the surgical staples within your hair after 10 to 12 days.

You'll have some redness at the suture line starting about two weeks after surgery, when hair emerges from the follicles buried beneath the hairline incision (fig. 11-9). The growing hair will slowly work its way through your hairline over the next few weeks. For several months, you'll also have some numbness, variable sensation, and occasional itchiness on your scalp behind the incision, but everything will gradually return to normal.

None of our patients has had infection, permanent weakness or paralysis of the forehead, or permanent hair loss. Only two patients had telogen (temporary hair loss) for a millimeter or two along the hairline. It went away completely. Most important, because of our special closure techniques, our patients haven't had a visible scar or complaints about the incision. All of our patients have been able to wear their hair pulled straight back and style it however they wished.

Results of the Forehead Lift

The forehead lift removes the excess skin which causes wrinkling in your forehead and raises the position of your eyebrows to make you look younger and more energetic. In achieving this result, however, we always caution patients not to fall into believing that "more is better." For example, we always leave the lowest forehead wrinkle untouched because it helps animate your eyebrows and gives you a natural expression. In addition, we never try to eliminate all movement of your forehead. That would give you an unnatural, "doll-like" appearance, instead of the natural, more youthful look we're seeking.

The most important concern in trying to achieve this youthful look is the final position of your eyebrows

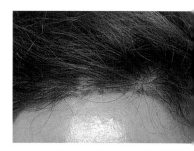

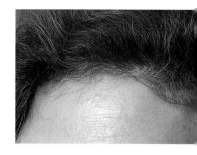

Fig. 11-9a (top). Close-up of hairline after forehead lift. The redness at the suture line is present for several weeks as the hair grows through and in front of this incision.

Fig. 11-9b (above). Same patient several weeks after surgery. Hair has grown through and in front of the hairline incision.

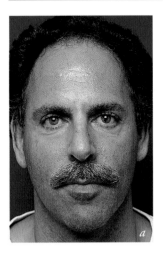
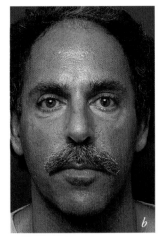
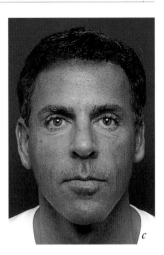

Fig. 11-10a. Pre-operative view of patient with frontal baldness and low eyebrows which give heavy, full appearance to upper eyelids.

Fig. 11-10b. Post-operative view of patient after forehead lift with incision in bald frontal scalp.

Fig. 11-10c. Several weeks later, with a Fleming/Mayer Flap rotated to eliminate frontal baldness.

after surgery. We always slightly overcorrect the brow position because the eyebrows will relax over a few weeks. This relaxed position will leave you looking far less tired, sad, or angry — and perfectly natural.

Usually, the forehead lift improves not only the drooping of the eyebrows but also the problem of excess skin on the upper eyelids, which changes our appearance with age. If there is any residual excess skin of the upper eyelids, it can be removed three to four months after the lift. If properly done, the forehead lift is an extremely safe and rewarding procedure. The keys are careful planning before the operation and meticulous surgical technique.

If you're considering hair-replacement surgery, you certainly want more hair, but, you also want to look better (fig. 11-10). The ideal time to correct the heavy, tired appearance that comes with forehead wrinkles and low eyebrows is before hair-replacement surgery. The incision for a forehead lift is within the bald skin that will be eliminated during hair replacement surgery, so it's better to do the forehead lift before rather than after the procedure to replace your hair. Anyone who is consulting a physician about hair replacement should always simultaneously consider a forehead lift.

12.
Tissue Expansion

During the last 10 years, the medical community has made great advances using tissue expansion in plastic surgery, including breast reconstruction, scalp reconstruction, and treatment of scars and burns. Tissue expanders slowly stretch the skin in much the same way that pregnancy stretches a woman's abdomen, essentially creating "new" skin for surgical procedures. Expansion is particularly useful in reconstructing damaged scalp or treating male-pattern baldness because it creates additional hair-bearing skin, which we can use to replace bald skin removed during a scalp reduction or to increase the size of a hair flap.

Although expansion isn't necessary for most balding patients undergoing flap surgery, it does offer many advantages, especially for people with tight scalps, prior punch grafting, or small areas of donor hair. As long as their hair has normal density, these otherwise marginal candidates can undergo tissue expansion and then--at the time the expanders are removed--have a scalp reduction or flap surgery.

For extensive bald areas, especially to cover male-pattern baldness, we can place an expander on either side of the head and make the scalp much larger before doing scalp reductions and flap surgery. For most cosmetic hair replacement surgery, however, we place only one expander at a time to lessen trauma to the scalp.

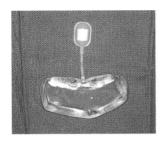

Fig. 12-1. Expander includes an inflatable balloon, connecting tube, and the small self-sealing port for injections of saline (saltwater). The entire apparatus is placed under the skin.

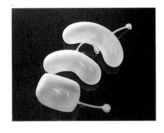

Fig. 12-2. Type A (top) is a larger sausage-shaped expander for Fleming/Mayer Flaps. Type B (middle) is a shorter version of the sausage-shaped expander used for shorter flaps and scalp reductions. Type C (bottom) is a small rectangular expander used to expand hair-bearing scalp for flaps based at the top of the temple (see Chapter 13).

Usually, one expander is also much less noticeable to others, and hair length and styling better camouflage a single expander.

As you can see in the illustration, the expander itself has three parts: a small, self-sealing port for injections of saline (saltwater) solution, a connecting tube, and an inflatable, silicone-rubber balloon (fig. 12-1). Expanders are available in different sizes and shapes. Depending on their purpose, they can be round, rectangular, square, or curving like a sausage.

Three types of expanders work especially well for male-pattern baldness (fig. 12-2). The larger sausage-shaped expander (type A) has the perfect length and shape for long Fleming/Mayer flaps. Type B is a shorter version of the sausage, suited for shorter flaps and scalp reductions. And the smaller, rectangular type C is used to expand hair-bearing scalp for flaps based at the top of the temple.

The Expansion Process

If we decide you need tissue expansion, we use a safe, straightforward procedure to place the expandable balloon under your hair-bearing scalp on the side of your head. All of the expander is under the scalp, and nothing shows above the skin. You'll need only local anesthesia for this surgery. We won't allow any of the balloon to be under bald skin because we want to avoid stretching the bald area. We locate the injection port away from the balloon so there is no risk of puncturing the balloon when injecting saline solution through the scalp and into the port. After inserting the expander, we close the incision and apply dressings. You'll take antibiotics after this operation to avoid infection, as well as medication for the first 24 hours to control light to moderate pain and swelling.

Once the expander is in place, we typically inject just enough saltwater solution through the port to make the expansion area slightly firm and prevent any spaces under the scalp. At this point, the expander places no pressure on the skin. You then wait 10 to 14 days before beginning the expansion process.

Because each injection of solution fills only five to 10 percent of the expander's volume, you'll need multiple injections to expand your hair-bearing scalp. If you have a willing relative or friend, he or she can quickly learn how to do these injections two times per week over six to eight weeks, eliminating the inconvenience of office visits. The ease of injections is important to many of our patients from other locations around the world. Although you may feel some discomfort after the first few injections, you can easily control it with medication and by limiting the amount of saline injected.

If you need to travel or conduct business during the expansion process, it's possible temporarily to remove part of the fluid from the expander for cosmetic reasons and then reinflate it later. Although this interruption delays completion, it makes expansion more flexible and acceptable to some patients. Given the advantages of tissue expansion, it's important to make necessary adjustments. Once tissue expansion is complete, we remove the expander at the time of a planned scalp reduction, reconstruction, or flap surgery.

Potential Concerns

Although tissue expansion is quite safe, it's important to consider possible concerns about the process to make sure you're prepared for it. Some patients initially resist the idea of having an expander placed beneath the scalp, especially for cosmetic hair replacement. Those who need reconstructive surgery are more motivated because the result will eliminate scars, burns, or other noticeable defects. However, if you have a very tight scalp, a small area of growing hair, or scarring from punch grafting, we must point out that the advantages of expansion are too great to resist. Many people are able to overcome their concern when they recognize that expansion leads to fewer overall surgeries and often makes hair replacement possible.

Sometimes, people are concerned about whether expansion is painful. We've talked about the moderate discomfort associated with putting the expander in place. This pain is slight to moderate and is controlled with medication. We have done many of these procedures on children, and they often take no medication.

In addition to these two concerns, most patients want to know how the expander will affect them cosmetically, how it will alter normal activities, and whether it can cause any complications. Let's consider some of these common questions now.

Is the Expander Noticeable?

For the first few weeks during expansion, swelling of the scalp is slight and unnoticeable. But in the last week or two the expander becomes large, so people who have short hair and large expanders will find it difficult to camouflage the expanded area. To conceal the expansion, we recommend that our patients simply grow their hair longer. By styling their longer hair, they are able to work right up to the time of scalp reduction or flap surgery with little cosmetic concern. We do many professionals — including doctors, lawyers, and celebrities — who continue with their normal daily routines.

What Happens to the Expanded Skin?

Although temporary microscopic changes occur, the skin is unchanged in outward appearance and sensation. Sometimes the shock of expansion causes the hair to thin because of an increased number of hairs in the telogen stage described in Chapter One, but it returns to normal in a few weeks.

Will I Have Trouble Sleeping?

You can sleep on an expander without causing any harm, but most people adjust by sleeping more often on the other side. If you have expanders on both sides at the same time, you may have a bit more trouble sleeping, but this is a minor complaint.

Can I Exercise Normally?

You must stop exercising for the first two or three weeks to avoid jarring the expander under the scalp. After that, exercises which don't damage the expander are fine, except for very strenuous activities and contact sports. You can jog or lift weights, but can't exert yourself intensely, as in training for competitive sports.

Are There Any Complications?

The complication rate for tissue expansion is very low among experienced plastic surgeons, and complications cause only minor inconvenience. Hematoma, or unwanted swelling under the skin, can occur with leakage from an artery or blood vessel. At worst, this condition might require removal of the expander, a brief office procedure to solve the problem, and reinsertion of the expander. But hematoma is extremely rare. Infection is possible when placing the expander under the scalp, but we prevent it by making sure you receive antibiotics after placement of an expander. If infection occurs (less than one-half percent of the time), the expander may have to be removed and replaced later.

Occasional leaks in the expander balloon and port used to be a problem. Modern methods and materials have solved this problem in the expander itself. Infrequently, the self-sealing port may develop a small leak under pressure, which requires removal and replacement of the port. In our practice, friends of patients occasionally used to damage the port while injecting saline. Now we use expanders with larger ports and are careful to explain this possibility to whoever is doing the injections, so it is a rare complication.

Advantages of Tissue Expansion

The greatest advantage of using expanders is that they create large amounts of "new" hair-bearing scalp. They also allow a surgeon to do in two procedures (expander placement and removal) what used to require several operations. Previously, in patients with ex-

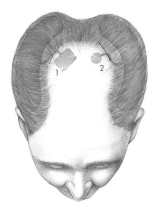

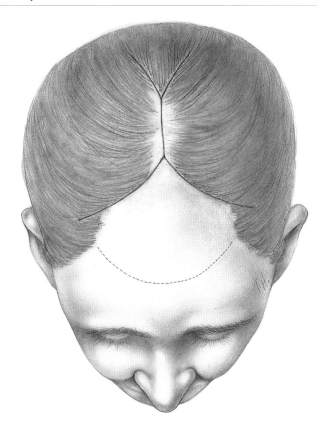

Fig. 12-3a (above). Bilateral tissue expanders placed before scalp reduction. Different sized ports (1 & 2) for injection of the saline. The interrupted dark lines show the incision for placement of expanders.

Fig. 12-3b (right). After removal of the expander, the baldness in the mid-portion of the scalp has been reduced. The frontal baldness is unchanged after a scalp reduction, so we must treat it with punch graft transplantation or flap surgery.

tremely tight scalps, a surgeon might have needed several scalp reductions, removing small amounts of bald skin with each procedure.

The advantage of expansion over standard scalp reductions is not as great in patients with normal scalp elasticity. Those who do have elastic scalps can choose two or three reductions instead of expansion. But those with inelastic scalps don't have this option. Tissue expansion can have an advantage over scalp reduction for people with marginal hair density, because we can expand areas of dense hair while not stretching an area of bald scalp or sparse hair (fig. 12-3). Scalp reductions tend to stretch all areas of the scalp equally to close up the removed section of skin.

Tissue expansion combined with scalp reduction is much better than hair transplantation when covering large areas of baldness (figs. 12-4). Expansion stretches

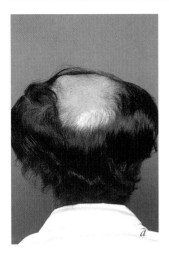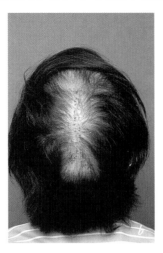

Fig. 12-4a. Patient with large bald area of central scalp and crown. The patient has limited donor scalp because he previously had extensive punch graft transplants to the frontal scalp. The expanders are in place on both sides of the scalp.

Fig. 12-4b. Patient after removal of the expanders and scalp reduction surgery. The grafts are seen in the frontal scalp. The size of the bald area has dramatically decreased, and we will treat the remaining area with punch graft transplantation.

hair-bearing scalp uniformly, with no tufting or other changes in hair texture. Stretched skin also has a strong blood supply and excellent hair growth, so it doesn't temporarily lose hair or depend on careful placement of hundreds of tiny grafts, as transplantation does.

When used with flap surgery, expansion allows us to take the flap from scalp with the densest hair. We place an expander having the same shape as the flap along the entire side and back of the donor scalp (fig. 12-5), expand the skin, and then do the two delays before removing the expander and rotating the flap into its final position. An expander increases the flap width by one-fourth to one-third over what is possible without expansion. It can also keep the flap surgery from raising the hairline behind the ear, a concern for patients with a small donor area. Finally, expansion decreases operating time, recovery time, and complications because the looser skin is easier to work with and to close under less tension (fig. 12-6).

Disadvantages of Tissue Expansion

We've talked about the need for two operations to place and remove the expander, as well as the cosmetic problems of trying to conceal expansion during the last two weeks. From the surgeon's point of view, however, the greatest disadvantage of tissue expansion is that it

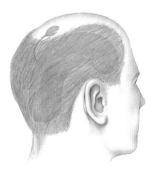

Fig. 12-5. Side view of Fleming/ Mayer tissue expander in place. The dark interrupted line at the fringe shows the incision for placement of the expander. The irregular lines show the future design of the Fleming/Mayer Flap to be used after expansion is complete.

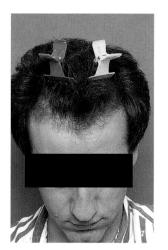 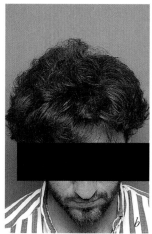 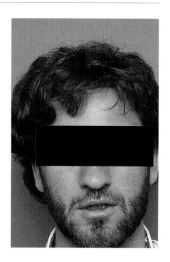

Fig. 12-6a. Pre-operative view of a patient with front hair loss. Sausage-shaped expander was used before Fleming/Mayer Flap rotation.

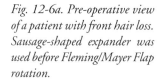

Fig. 12-6b and 12-6c. Patient six days after rotation of Fleming/Mayer Flap with complete elimination of baldness.

can't cover baldness of the frontal scalp on its own. As figure 12-3b shows, even with tissue expansion, a scalp reduction leaves a "piece of pie" defect in the frontal scalp to midscalp. Although patients can style hair over this area to some extent, we must re-establish the hairline with either punch grafts or flaps.

Despite these disadvantages, tissue expansion is a very important addition to the tools available for hair replacement. It gives us more flexibility in dealing with baldness from injury or natural processes. Although not a "cure" for complete baldness in itself, it works superbly with scalp reduction and flap surgeries. Tissue expanders also provide gratifying results when dealing with difficult cases requiring reconstructive surgery (see Chapter 14).

13.
Other Flaps Used for Scalp Surgery

This chapter and the next pick up two categories of "odds and ends." Our discussion of other types of flaps in this chapter or of reconstructive surgery in Chapter 14 isn't necessary to most readers seeking advice about baldness, but it may cover a special problem that applies to you.

The "Short" (Temporo-Parietal) Flap

With the advent of long flaps in 1975, others began to modify them by making them shorter, narrower, and random (not connected to an axis of skin for rotation). These shorter flaps lend themselves to repairing smaller areas of baldness and may sometimes be necessary if a person doesn't have enough donor hair for a full-length flap. To further improve their design, we've modified short flaps to include an axis incorporating the superficial temporal artery for better blood supply and created the irregular hairline described in earlier chapters. Despite these improvements, however, we don't usually recommend them; their narrow, short design doesn't allow them to replace a large bald area or baldness at the mid-scalp or crown for patients with Class III baldness.

Flap Design — A single short flap doesn't extend across the entire width of your forehead. The first flap is designed to extend beyond the center of your forehead, if possible (fig. 13-1). The second flap is shorter still, so

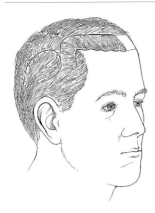

Fig. 13-1. Inferiorly based short flap as modified by Fleming and Mayer. Flap has been rotated to the frontal scalp and the donor area closed. The irregular dark line shows the location for the future (second) flap.

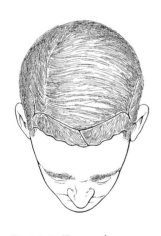

Fig. 13-2. Two weeks or more after doing the first flap, we can take a second flap from the opposite side to complete the hairline. If a large area of baldness remains behind these flaps, scalp reductions and hair transplants will be necessary.

it's even less likely to lose hair or have skin damage at the tip. However, it's made long enough to join the first flap. To prevent a partline from being visible where the two flaps meet, we design them to dovetail together at an angle of 45 to 60 degrees (fig. 13-2). The flap comes from the scalp over your ear, following a gentle curve from near your temples to the side of your head. We keep it well within your donor area throughout its length and make it about an inch wide.

Flap Procedure — Because this flap doesn't need a delay before transposing it to replace part of your bald scalp, we can lift it from the donor area, rotate it, and suture it into the recipient area in one operation. Otherwise, the technique — including closure of your donor area — is much the same as for a long flap. As we're placing the first flap into position, we also mark your hairline for the second flap (on the other side).

We move the second flap two weeks after the first. Although both flaps could be transposed at the same time, we wait mainly because doing so allows the scalp to regain some elasticity before we make more incisions on the other side of your head. Waiting two weeks allows us to adjust the length of the second flap in case damage occurs at the end of the first one.

Just as for the long flap, a dog-ear is produced when the flap rotates on itself to create your new hairline. We can remove this twist of skin about six weeks after rotating your flap. In most cases, however, it goes away on its own within two to three months.

Dressings and postoperative care are essentially the same as for the long flap. You can expect to be off work for six days, after which you can resume all activities except heavy exercise. About a month later, you can go back to your normal routine.

Use of Short Flaps — These short flaps obviously will not provide as much coverage as the Fleming/Mayer Flap because flaps from both sides of the head are used to eliminate only frontal baldness. Any remaining baldness behind the flaps can be surgically treated only

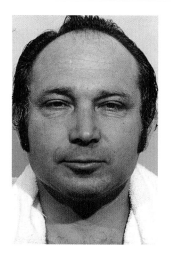 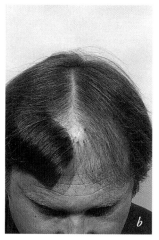 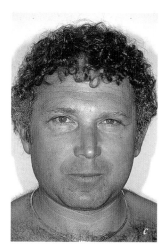

with reductions and transplants (fig. 13-3). Usually baldness does extend beyond the frontal one inch of the scalp, making short flaps a poor choice for most men with male-pattern baldness.

Two special circumstances may call for short flaps. First, we can use them to replace some Class III baldness when your scalp is too scarred, inelastic, or short to allow long flaps. Second, you may choose short flaps if you don't have enough hair for a long flap and are committed to wearing a hair addition. We use short flaps to provide a superior hairline for the hair addition because it's hard to achieve a natural look along the hairline of hairpieces (fig. 13-4). But you can't change your mind about wearing a hair addition after having short-flap surgery for this purpose. The short flap doesn't replace enough of your baldness on its own to provide an aesthetically pleasing result.

The relative simplicity of short flaps does appeal to some people. But if you choose this approach, you can't get long flaps later because the donor areas on both sides of the head have already been used.

Other Flaps

Axial Flaps — An axial flap is simply one based on a known artery. We can design many different kinds of axial flaps depending on the patient's needs. They're

Fig. 13-3a. Forty-two-year-old patient with frontal baldness before his operation.

Fig. 13-3b. View showing one flap in place. A second flap is rotated approximately two weeks after the first.

Fig. 13-3c. Three months after rotation of two short (temporal parietal) flaps. One scalp reduction behind the flaps totally eliminated his baldness.

used mainly for reconstructive work or to replace small bald areas. Other than the long and short flaps already described, the two most common are occipital (back of the head) and postauricular (behind the ear).

Occipital flaps have been used to replace crown baldness. These flaps are designed so the attachment is down low in the back of the neck instead of over the ear as in a long flap. But we believe a conventional long flap can handle crown baldness better because its hair direction is backward over the crown. The postauricular flap is attached behind the ear. It's rather short, so it would rarely be used for pattern baldness unless other flaps were impossible. Its most common application is in traumatic or reconstructive problems, such as burns or scarring. The design would depend on the location, size, and form of the defect.

Random Flaps — It's possible to take small flaps from other (random) locations in your scalp, without basing them on an artery, and then to place them wherever they're needed. In other words, we would simply elevate a section of hair-bearing scalp and move it to an area of bald or scarred scalp.

One advantage with these flaps in treating baldness at the hairline is that we can "turn them around" so the hair would grow forward, as it did before hair loss occurred (fig. 13-5, 13-6). Unfortunately, many disadvantages outweigh this slight advantage. Added prob-

Fig. 13-4a. Patient with extensive baldness and inadequate donor hair to perform the Fleming/Mayer Flaps. He had numerous reductions and transplants before coming to us. The patient was committed to wearing a hair addition.

Fig. 13-4b. View after two short (temporal parietal) Flaps to establish a natural hairline with his own hair.

Fig. 13-4c. Hair addition in place after short flap surgery.

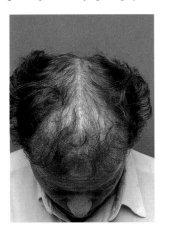
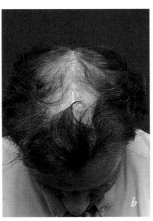
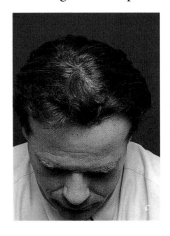

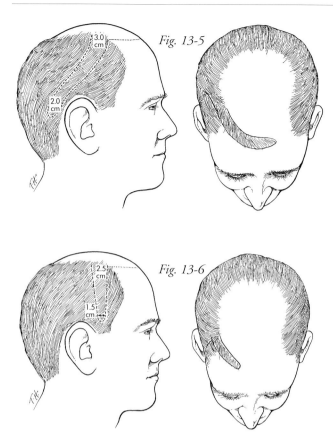

Fig. 13-5. Flap taken from the side of the scalp and based superiorly near the fringe. The irregular dark line represents the design of the narrow flap. The vertical scar which is present after removal of the flap is difficult to conceal. This flap does not reach the opposite side except in unusual circumstances.

Fig. 13-6. Flap from the temple based superiorly at the fringe. The dark irregular line shows the design of the flap. This small flap eliminates only part of the very large bald area.

Fig. 13-7 (below). Design of the superiorly based temporal flap as modified by Fleming and Mayer. Design and placement of Fleming/Mayer type C tissue expander are shown. Note the flap extending beyond the midline. A second flap will be done from the opposite side.

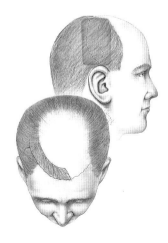

lems may occur because there is no artery within the base of the flap. More skin damage is likely because this flap doesn't have an axial blood supply, and hair quality is poorer than with a long flap because it's taken from thinner areas in front of the ear. Most important, this random flap is very short and narrow, so a person with Class III baldness would still have large areas to cover with reductions or punch grafting. Incision scars tend to spread and are more visible in this finer hair. Finally, these flaps rarely reach the midline, so it's very difficult to complete the hairline without using tissue expansion (see Chapter 12).

Despite these disadvantages, you could use this procedure if you have only mild frontal baldness that won't progress; high, full hair toward the front of your temples; good hair quality in front of your ear. You

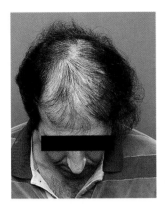

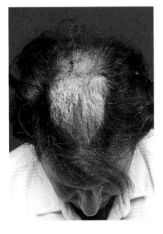

Fig. 13-8a. Patient who had previous punch graft transplantation for treatment of frontal baldness at 45 years of age and later had significant hair loss behind and between the grafts as well as into the crown. Pre-operative view shows exposed grafts and exten-sive thinning into the crown.

Fig. 13-8b. Same patient after rotation of second flap. Reductions and punch grafting will reduce the residual baldness in the center of the scalp and the crown.

should also be willing to accept tissue expansion, which is almost always necessary.

If you meet all of these conditions, we would first place an expander beneath the scalp at your temple (see Chapter 12) to increase your donor area (fig. 13-7). After about two months of expansion, we can mark off your hairline and do the flap procedure.

The person in figure 13-8 underwent this kind of procedure and got an excellent hairline from it. But when we tie the flap hair and see the bald area behind it, we recognize that scalp reduction and punch grafting will still be necessary. When compared with the results you've seen with the Fleming/Mayer Flap, you can understand why we seldom use this type of flap.

Free Flaps — A free flap is a flap in which the artery within its axial base is cut and then resutured into an artery within the recipient scalp. Although some surgeons have used free flaps in hair replacement or reconstruction, we believe they have three major disadvantages that recommend against them. They require the surgeon to reconnect tiny blood vessels under a microscope in order to supply blood to the flap. Otherwise, a large part of the flap may be lost to necrosis. This high risk of failure makes them unacceptable to us and our patients. They also require considerable time and therefore are very expensive.

If free flaps gave vastly better results in hair direction or general appearance when compared to long flaps, they might be worth the risk and cost. Unfortunately, they don't.

Although some of the flaps mentioned in this chapter have a place in very specialized hair-replacement surgery, none substitutes effectively for the Fleming/Mayer Flap discussed in Chapter 10. But you may be one of those rare people who are unable to have standard flap surgery. If so, knowing what kinds of results to expect from these alternatives will enable you to decide whether to rely on them, on transplants, or on a hair addition to replace your lost hair.

14.
Reconstructive Surgery

Most people find it comforting to know that surgical procedures are available to treat defects of the scalp existing at birth or caused by injury, burns, disease, or previous medical treatment. If you have bald areas from any of these causes, surgical solutions would vary depending on blood supply and other characteristics. Because we can't discuss here every possible combination of injury, defect size and shape, and location, we'll simply share with you our basic approach and philosophy regarding reconstruction of scalp defects.

We use seven main types of reconstructive surgery to repair scalp defects:

1. Simple removal of small areas of alopecia (baldness)
2. Hair transplantation (including micrografts)
3. Removing alopecia scars and closing with Z-plasties
4. Scalp reduction
5. Tissue expansion
6. Small transposition flaps
7. Fleming-Mayer flaps

We've discussed most of these procedures in separate chapters, so we'll limit ourselves here to ways they are particularly effective for reconstruction.

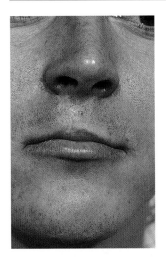

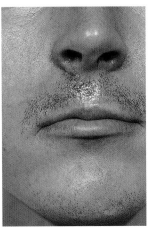

Fig. 14-1a. Pre-operative view of patient with a traumatic scar of upper lip referred to us for hair transplantation to his upper lip.

Fig. 14-1b. View at three months after the operation. We simply revised the scar and excised the bald area without transplantation.

Simple Removal

We can usually make incisions on each side of small bald or scarred areas, remove the skin containing the defect, and suture together the edges created by the incisions (fig. 14-1). To get the best hair growth, we must bevel these incisions parallel to the hair follicles. Whenever hair is growing in the same direction on both sides of the defect, this simple procedure is all that's necessary. If hair growth diverges noticeably, we can transplant these areas with punch grafts containing one or two hairs (micrografts), as discussed in Chapter 9, or use the Z-plasties discussed later in this chapter.

Hair Transplantation

Transplantation is usually our last choice for most reconstructive problems because of the poor blood supply in the recipient area. Although grafts will grow in scar tissue, often the yield per graft is less than in an area of normal circulation. Because of this decreased yield, as well as poor hair density, changes in texture, and the length of time needed to complete the procedure, we seldom use transplantation.

We do use punch grafts in scarred areas of the lip or eyebrow which are too large to allow removal without distorting the surrounding tissue (fig. 14-2). We would also do punch grafting if other procedures in this chapter were impossible because of some medical condition or were unacceptable to a particular patient.

Removing Scars and Closing with Z-Plasty

Often, small areas of scarring from injury, tumors, or medical procedures have hair that "wants to part" because it diverges on either side of the defect. This divergence is even more marked if the area is wide or if it results from one or more scalp reductions. Simple incisions and removal won't improve the scar because divergence will occur again along the new closure. If we remove a large amount of bald or scarred skin, the middle and back parts of the scalp will have hair growing in

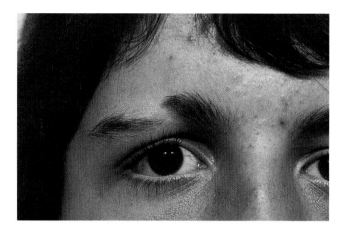

Fig. 14-2a. Pre-operative view of spontaneous baldness in the middle of the eyebrow which developed when the patient was five years old.

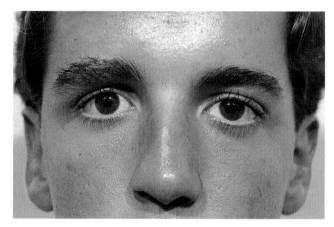

Fig. 14-2b. Same patient after twenty punch grafts.

opposite directions on either side of the incision. This growth creates an unnatural part down the center of the head. Burns or injury can cause the same problem in other parts of the scalp.

As long as the hair next to the scar has good density, we can excise the scarred skin and then do several Z-plasties to redirect the hair across the area. A Z-plasty is a zig-zag incision which allows us to bring hair from each side of the scar and place it in an irregular pattern across the area of the original incision. As a result, the original straight scar is made into an irregular incision hidden by the alternating direction of hair growth across the area.

The patient in figure 14-3 is a 36-year-old man who came to our office after having 400 punch grafts placed

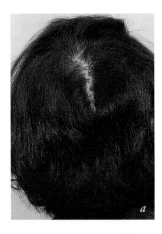

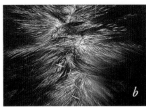

Fig. 14-3a. Patient seen in our office after 400 hair transplants to the frontal scalp and scalp reductions. Unnatural "axe-like" scar with parting of the hair after scalp reductions. Hair growing in divergent directions on each side of the scar.

Fig. 14-3b. Excision of scar and multiple Z-plasties have changed hair direction, eliminated the divergent growth pattern, and brought thick hair into the defect created by excising the scar.

Fig. 14-3c. With its direction of growth changed, the hair lies naturally over the incision.

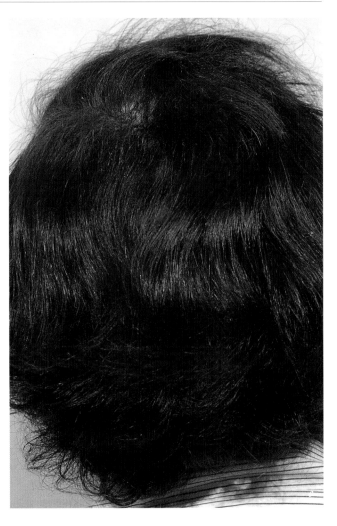

to establish a new hairline and scalp reductions behind the frontal area. He was unhappy with the "part" toward the top back of his head. We removed the scar and did several Z-plasties while changing the hair direction and thereby eliminating the divergent hair growth. Because thick hair is now growing in the previously scarred area, the patient doesn't have to resort to careful hairstyling to camouflage the scar.

Scalp Reduction

Scalp reductions allow us to remove even rather large scarred areas and replace them with healthy, hair-

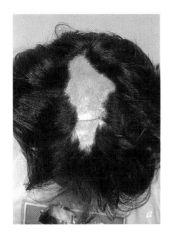 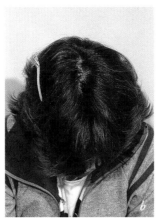

Fig. 14-4a. Pre-operative view of 12-year-old patient with thermal burns of the scalp treated with skin grafts.

Fig. 14-4b. Same patient after two scalp reductions to eliminate the scarring.

bearing skin in much the same way as we've discussed for baldness in Chapter Eight. Assuming the patient has an elastic scalp, we can remove part of the scarred skin, stretch and advance healthy tissue into the area, and close the defect with sutures. Depending on the size of the scarring, scalp laxity will return and additional reductions can be done about 10-12 weeks apart.

An example of this technique for scalp reconstruction involved the 12-year-old patient in Figure 14-4. She had scalp burns which had been skin grafted and was referred to us for reconstruction. During each of three scalp reductions, we moved the healthy scalp on each side toward the midline of her head, removed excess skin, and advanced the scalp from the back of her head forward and toward the midline. The patient returned to school the day after each surgical procedure.

Tissue Expansion

Many patients have tight scalps with little or no potential for reduction. Their only choices for surgery are punch grafting (Chapter Nine) or tissue expansion (Chapter 12) with scalp reductions or transposition flaps. Often, these patients have scarring or injury, or both, in the arteries of the scalp, which may keep us from using transposition flaps. In this case, we prefer expansion and reductions over punch grafting, which has the limitations mentioned earlier as well as relatively

Fig. 14-5a. Four-year-old girl with severe scarring that resulted from an automobile accident. Skin grafts are in place over the injured area. Pre-operative view.

Fig. 14-5b. Expander in place and fully expanded before scalp advancement.

Fig. 14-5c. Scalp baldness has been eliminated after removing the expander and advancing the normal, hair-bearing skin. The remaining defects are outlined with an ink pen. Expanders were then placed in the cheek and forehead.

Fig. 14-5d. Immediately after removal of these expanders and excision of forehead and cheek scarring.

Fig. 14-5e and 14-5f. Final post-operative appearance.

Fig. 14-5g. Hair parted showing normal density.

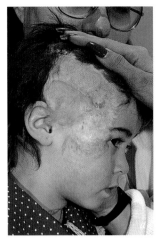
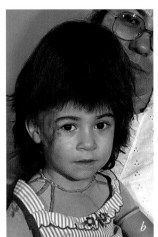
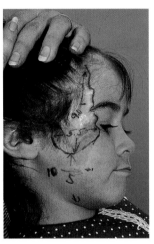
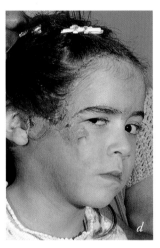
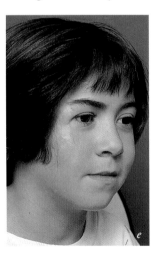
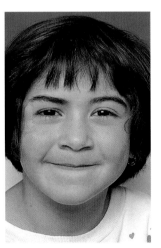
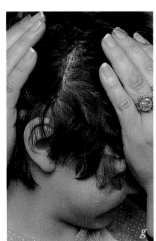

poor results in areas of reduced blood circulation (scarring). Typically, we use one expander at a time if we can completely remove a scarred area and replace it with expanded hair-bearing scalp having good density. One expander is also best when the patient has two separate problem areas located next to one another, so we can avoid enlarging or putting strain on the scarred area. Here, we expand one donor area at a time and alternate with reduction to remove the problem scalp in stages.

At times, it's possible to expand two separate areas of donor scalp simultaneously, so we can remove a larger scarred area while maintaining enough hair density over the two donor locations.

The patient in Figure 14-5 was a four-year-old girl who was struck by a car and dragged along the pavement. She had multiple skin grafts and was then referred to us for reconstructive surgery. As you can see in the figure, she had a large scalp defect, with scarring extending onto the forehead, the right cheek, and the right ear. The young girl had a very tight scalp, so tissue expansion was necessary. We placed a large expander underneath the surrounding hair-bearing scalp. After the skin was stretched for five weeks, we removed the expander and advanced the surrounding normal scalp to replace the scarring.

Some scars remained on the right cheek and right forehead, so we placed expanders in these areas to stretch this skin. After that skin was stretched, we removed nearly all of the scarring.

Another of our patients was a young woman who had an allergic reaction to medication placed on the scalp to treat lice infection when she was seven years old. As a result, she lost hair in the crown and center of her scalp. She had several reductions and hair transplants before our first consultation, so the scalp was very tight. We placed tissue expanders on each side of her head to stretch the normal hair-bearing skin. After removing the expanders, we excised all of the scarred scalp and advanced the normal scalp into its place.

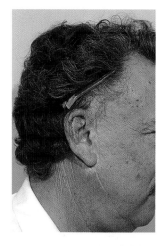

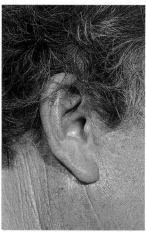

Fig. 14-6a (top). Pre-operative appearance of a patient who previously had a facelift that eliminated the sideburn. He was referred to us for reconstructive surgery.

Fig. 14-6b (above). Appearance after rotating a flap based in the upper part of the temple and reestablishing the sideburn.

Transposition Flaps

These flaps, discussed in more detail in Chapters 10 and 13, are often useful in reconstructing of the frontal scalp. They allow us to bring hair-bearing tissue from the sides and back of the head to the frontal scalp, maintain good hair direction, and make incisions used to place the flap undetectable. In contrast, scalp reductions (with or without tissue expansion) don't work well for frontal reconstruction, because the hair in areas next to these scalp defects often is sparse, won't "reach" to the front hairline or temples, or grows in the wrong direction. Reductions which advance scalp into the frontal area also may leave a visible scar along the front hairline.

Small Transposition Flaps — We can use small flaps based along the temporal artery to reconstruct eyebrows, sideburns, or small defects of the scalp. For example, patients are often referred to us who have had facelift procedures that raised or eliminated the sideburns. In this case, a temporal flap is useful to re-establish the normal distribution of hair. The type of flap used depends on the tightness or elasticity of the scalp, the amount of donor hair available at the temple, and the location of any scars in the temporal hair created by previous procedures. If no scars are at the temples, we can take a random flap, suture it in place to form a sideburn, and directly close the defect at the original location of the flap. If a scar is present, we may need to base a longer flap with a pedicle and axis in the upper part of the temple behind the scar. We would then rotate the flap forward, suture it into place to form the sideburn, and close the resulting defect behind the scar (see Figure 14-6).

A final category of small flap includes those we can take from any place on the scalp to repair small defects. These flaps are usually random, having no axis or pedicle. They may sometimes be based on an artery to improve blood supply. These types of flaps are often necessary to treat scars in the frontal scalp, for cases in which scalp reductions aren't helpful.

Temporoparietal Flaps — The temporoparietal flap, taken from the donor hair at the temples and front side of the head, is longer than the flaps discussed above but shorter than the Fleming-Mayer (long) Flap discussed below. It may be based either lower in this area (nearer the top of the ear) or higher (nearer the partline). As discussed in Chapter 13, two short, temporoparietal flaps based on the lower part of this region can't remove the same amount of scar tissue replaced by a long flap. Thus, we seldom use them for reconstructive surgery, but we would use them in patients who:

1. Have a full head of hair and no possibility of future baldness, and who have scar tissue or baldness only along the front one inch of the hairline or other small frontal location.
2. Do not have a superficial temporal artery necessary for long flaps--usually because of a previous injury or surgery.
3. Have heavily punch-grafted donor areas, which would greatly increase the risk of hair or skin loss at the end of a long flap.

The patient in Figure 14-7 shows how this type of flap works in reconstructive surgery. He had received several sessions of punch grafting and had many scars in the frontal scalp. Heavy scarring was also present in the donor areas, which would have increased the risk of hair or skin loss at the end of a long flap. Because this patient had established baldness with little expected future loss, we decided to remove the scar tissue using two short flaps. Scalp reductions wouldn't have replaced the frontal scars with hair-bearing scalp, and the patient didn't want more punch grafting. As you can see in the figure, styling is a bit more difficult with two short flaps than with a long flap but much easier than with punch-grafted hair. The patient has better hair density, natural texture, and no noticeable "corn-row" appearance.

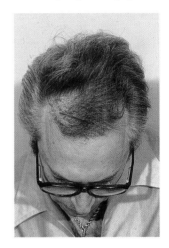

Fig. 14-7a (below). Patient had extensive punch grafting to his frontal scalp before we saw him and wasn't satisfied with the density achieved. His donor scalp was heavily scarred from harvesting of his hair transplants.

Fig. 14-7b (bottom). Same patient after placement of two short temporoparietal flaps.

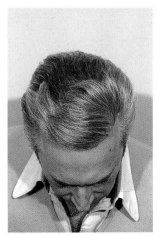

The Fleming-Mayer Flap

The long flap is best for most reconstructive scalp surgery. It is used frequently for reconstructing the frontal scalp but also works well in the midscalp or crown. As mentioned earlier, scalp reductions don't bring hair into the frontal scalp, so we must use either punch grafts or flaps to reconstruct this area. But poor blood supply in scarred scalp causes the yield of hair in each punch graft to be much lower than normal. This reduced yield and other relative disadvantages of punch grafting (see Chapters Nine and 10) make punch grafting a distant second choice in reconstruction of the scalp. Only long flaps can remove considerable scarring and immediately replace it with dense growing hair that gives a person natural texture, uniformity, and ease of styling.

In a surgeon's eyes, the results of reconstructive surgery usually don't match the ideal results of carefully planned original procedures, but they can be very satisfying. The examples in this chapter should show you that difficult, even apparently hopeless, scalp problems can often be overcome with effective surgical techniques. In fact, recent improvements in flap surgery and tissue expansion have brought these techniques into a new era. If you have problems of this type with your scalp, we strongly urge you to consult with a surgeon skilled in reconstructive scalp surgery.

15.
Choosing
a Doctor

Your first consultation with a doctor is very important to making decisions which lead to successful hair-replacement surgery. During that interview, you should get as much information as you can about your prospective surgeon and the kinds of operations available to you. Because most doctors don't do all hair replacement procedures, you can choose to find one who does or visit more than one surgeon to learn all of your alternatives. A reputable doctor will ask enough questions about you to ensure you're a good candidate for the recommended procedure. Complete information, combined with proper motivation and expectations on your part, normally leads to a much more satisfactory outcome.

Your doctor should be a physician with particular training in hair-replacement procedures. Your first step in finding the right surgeon is to take recommendations from family, friends, other doctors, or business associates who have had surgery themselves or know of someone who has undergone one of these procedures. Ask them how they located their surgeon, whether they're happy with the results and would return to the same surgeon for another procedure, and whether revisions (additional surgery) were necessary to achieve the proper result. You may also wish to ask about the cost.

If you can't find a physician through these kinds of recommendations, ask your family doctor or call medical schools or the medical society in your area. Although they won't endorse individual doctors, they will provide you with a list of names to choose from.

Asking the Right Questions

After you've selected two or three candidate surgeons, arrange an interview with each one and prepare to ask questions about the procedure, techniques the surgeon will use, recuperation time, possible complications, and so on. Ask about the doctor's qualifications and the preparation of those who may attend him. Any doctor with a good reputation and confidence in his professional ability will be happy to discuss results and qualifications. Of course, some tact is in order when asking about a doctor's abilities, but your health and appearance depend on your being persistent enough to discover what you need to know.

As a minimum, you should find out whether a physician has gone through a residency program to become qualified in his specialty. And look for certification in this specialty — a document that shows he has passed an examination given by his peers. Besides these formal qualifications, physicians should also be able to demonstrate their standing in the medical community by showing you they are members of your county's medical society or that they are affiliated with a hospital or medical school. These associations usually ensure that a physician's practice of medicine is consistent with professional standards.

Perhaps most important is to determine the physician's experience with hair transplants or flap surgery, as well as how involved he is personally with the procedure. Has he done enough transplants or flaps to make you confident in his skills and results? Does he do only the minimum surgery and turn over most of the procedure to assistants? Or does he do all of the surgery himself? Is he available to see you after the surgery, in case a problem arises? Combined with viewing photographs, videotapes, and actual patients, the answers to these questions should help you choose a surgeon who will meet your needs.

Because doctors don't do every step in a hair-replacement surgery, you should also make sure they have trained assistants to back them up. For example, assistants often handle cleaning and preparation of punch grafts after the doctor removes these grafts from the donor area. By asking questions about the assistants' qualifications and experience, you'll know whether you can expect professional service throughout the operation.

A less tangible but important part of your selection is compatibility of styles and personalities. In other words, your doctor's approach should make you comfortable and confident. If you like to have details on every aspect of surgery in advance, you'll be more comfortable with a physician who wants his patients to participate. When your doctor matches your expectations, your surgery will be much less stressful.

Finally, don't hesitate to get more than one medical opinion. A reputable doctor or clinic will avoid high-pressure tactics designed to keep you from consulting with others. By visiting different doctors, you'll also get a better idea of the results you can expect. Their judgments about the elasticity of your scalp or amount of donor hair available will influence your choice of procedure and its outcome. Hearing more than one doctor's opinion will reassure you or, at least, prepare you to make an informed decision.

Some people also seek a second opinion about the cost of surgery — a practice that makes sense within limits. Although the more expensive physician doesn't necessarily do a better job, hunting for bargains can lead to unsatisfactory, and even unfortunate, results. In most cases, because a good hair-replacement surgeon must have both medical expertise and artistic skill, you get what you pay for. If a skilled surgeon spends more time on a procedure, rather than turning over most of the work to assistants, your cost will go up. The smartest course is to balance your ability to pay against your expectations and then to choose the person who is likely to satisfy those expectations.

You should be especially careful of the "clinics" you may find heavily advertised in your daily newspaper and the doctors who work for them. Sometimes, non-medical salespeople run these clinics, recruiting customers and hiring physicians for "assembly-line" procedures. Because no special license is required for hair-replacement surgery, any medical doctor can do. Too often, a clinic will hire an inexperienced doctor who may even be "moonlighting" from another position. The doctor may be perfectly competent in his normal practice, but you want someone with surgical skill and an artist's understanding of your face and hairline. A good way to avoid surprises is to get the name, address, and phone number of the physician who will operate on you, so you can check on his credentials and experience.

Getting the Right Information

A good clinic will offer written information and before-and-after photographs for your review. Some will have videotapes available to more clearly illustrate procedures. You should also insist on meeting with patients who have had hair-replacement surgery--an excellent way to gather information and to see actual results. You should be able to learn about all the options available to you, not just the surgical procedure most often practiced by the clinic.

Written Information — As a prospective patient, you can expect information to flow both ways. Many doctors will ask you to fill out a cosmetic-surgery questionnaire, so they can learn more about you. They'll also give you brochures describing their hair-replacement techniques.

A cosmetic-surgery questionnaire asks you to answer "yes" or "no" to questions that make sure you have reasonable expectations for hair-replacement surgery. If you're reasonable and well motivated, you're much more likely to be satisfied with the results. If you're not asked for this kind of information before your consultation, consider carefully whether the doctor knows enough about you to meet your expectations.

A descriptive booklet should tell you about the advantages and disadvantages of all hair-replacement methods, as well as how you'd be suited for each one. It may describe how much discomfort you could have after an operation and how the surgery would limit your activities. Also important are potential complications, how much hair coverage you'll have during several stages of surgery, and the time necessary for cosmetic improvement. Finally, you should learn about the lab tests needed before your operation and how much everything will cost. If this information isn't in a booklet, be sure to ask about it during your consultation.

Viewing Photographs or Videotape — When you go in for your consultation, you should also be able to look at photographs of results. Surgeons will photograph patients before and after an operation. These photographs help them plan operations and assess their success, but they can also give you an inaccurate view of potential changes in your hair and scalp. For example, darker lighting in an "after" picture will create the impression that the hair is thicker than it really is. Or you may see a picture of a sparse crown, in which the head is tilted forward 15 degrees more than in the "before" picture. A slight amount of tilting creates the illusion of a much smaller bald spot, thus potentially exaggerating the effects of the hair-replacement surgery.

Even the best pictures can show you only the results for that moment. For example, because hair loss is progressive, results of hair transplants can be hidden by existing hair which hasn't yet fallen out within the transplanted area. The same view of this "completed result" taken a few years later may be less satisfactory, especially as more hair falls out behind the transplants. Always ask to see a patient who has completed the balding process and is now done with hair transplantation.

Finally, certain photographs depend on hair styling

to camouflage actual results. For example, curly or kinky hair can look ideal in photographs when in fact careful hair styling has produced this appearance. It's very important to see pictures with the hair parted to show tufting or "corn rows" (clumps of hair with spaces between them) and the density obtained. The results of hair-replacement surgery can be grossly misrepresented by not fully parting the hair, or by parting it in an area of thicker hair and using the remaining hair to cover extremely thin areas.

Because of the potential for misrepresenting hair-replacement surgery through photographs, we've done our best in this text to show clear, non-camouflaged results without hair being combed over (except in the hair-styling sections). Still, if you're trying to decide whether to have hair-replacement surgery, you should be particularly careful about using photographs as the sole basis for your judgment. Always try to see a videotape and to talk with actual patients before deciding which procedure best suits your needs.

Interviewing People Who Have Had Surgery — Happy patients are usually willing to show their results to other prospective patients, which is quite helpful and reassuring. Although we do all methods of hair replacement surgery, we especially like to use patients who have had flap surgery to demonstrate the uniform hair growth, excellent density, natural hair texture, and immediate outcome that you can obtain with flaps. Fifteen years ago, when flaps were little known, this was more important than today. Yet, because of the natural appearance after flap surgery, many people still aren't familiar with the results of this technique even when they see it daily.

Talking with patients is a very good way for you to see what a person looks like after surgery, as well as to ask questions about the experience itself. They can tell you how their expectations were met, how the surgery went, and what they experienced during the brief recuperation necessary for most hair-replacement procedures.

ACNE   An inflammation of the skin probably caused by testosterone (male hormone) levels and the sebaceous (oil) glands.   When excess oil clogs a pore or hair follicle, pimples often result.   Baldness treatments based on the theory that hair loss results from "clogged follicles" don't recognize that this "clogging" would cause acne and ingrown hairs on bald scalp.

ALDACTONE   A hypertension drug made by Searle and Company.   Like minoxidil (Rogaine), this drug may help stop hair loss or regrow hair.   Still being tested.

ALOPECIA   Aristotle coined this term in 384 B.C. to describe hair loss or baldness from any cause.   When used along with another word, it means the hair loss comes from a specific condition (e.g., Alopecia Prematura = premature baldness).

ALOPECIA AREATA   A dramatic form of hair loss in which smooth, circular patches of baldness suddenly appear.   Stress, immune-system problems, heredity, and other conditions can cause this loss, which is usually temporary.

ALOPECIA TOTALIS   Baldness in which all of the hair on the scalp falls out.   This is not male-pattern baldness, which maintains a fringe of hair around the sides and back of the head that never goes bald.

ALOPECIA UNIVERSALIS   A condition in which every hair on the body falls out.   It appears suddenly—like alopecia areata, and its causes aren't known.

5-ALPHA REDUCTASE   An enzyme produced in follicles genetically programmed for baldness.   When this enzyme is present, normal testosterone changes to dihydrotestosterone (DHT) in these follicles and launches the balding process.

AMINO ACIDS   Amino acids are groups of molecules that connect cells in building the human body. Cystine is an amino acid that gives hair its strength and stiffness, so normal amounts are necessary to the diet.   But adding amino acids to the diet or to lotions for the hair doesn't restore lost hair.

ANAGEN   Hair grows and sheds in three cycles: anagen, catagen, and telogen. Anagen is the growth stage, which lasts two to five years.

ANDROGEN   Male hormone.   Testosterone is the most powerful male hormone and is a player in male-pattern baldness.   Women normally produce small amounts of androgen, but increased production after menopause can lead to hair loss.   A number of baldness treatments under development are anti-androgens, which interfere with testosterone in the hair follicle.

ANDROGENETIC ALOPECIA   (See MALE-PATTERN BALDNESS.)

ANESTHETIC   An agent that produces insensitivity to pain or touch.   Local anesthetics are used in all forms of hair-replacement surgery.

ANTIBODIES   Substances produced by the body to defend itself from foreign "invaders."   An important part of immune-system research concerning the causes of baldness, antibodies may incorrectly attack hair follicles or substances.

AUTO-IMMUNE RESPONSE   Condition under which the body attempts to reject its own tissue. Caused when the immune system "misreads" the identity of a set of cells and sees them as invaders. This potential reason for baldness is now being researched.

BACITRACIN OINTMENT   An antibiotic cream which some doctors apply to the scalp after transplant surgery to help promote healing.

BIOTIN   Formerly called Vitamin H. It's produced by the human intestinal tract but is also one of the most common dietary supplements supposed to aid hair loss. Rare deficiencies in biotin do cause hair loss, but this loss has nothing to do with male-pattern baldness.

BONDING   (See FUSION.)

CASTRATION   Surgical removal of the testicles in the male and the ovaries in the female. Important to research on baldness because males castrated before puberty (eunuchs)—before they begin to produce testosterone in hair follicles—never go bald.

CATAGEN   The middle stage of hair growth—a transitional phase between the growing and resting phases. Although the hair isn't growing during this stage, it's still visible coming out of the follicle.

CHEMOTHERAPY   Cancer therapy with drugs that affect the entire body. Hair loss is a frequent side-effect.

CHOLINE   A water-soluble substance the liver needs to function. It's often added to B complex vitamins and found in baldness treatments, but there's no evidence that it can treat male-pattern baldness.

CICATRICIAL   Literally means scarring. Used with alopecia to describe a form of baldness that occurs because of scarring on the scalp, often from burns or accidents.

COLLAGEN   One of the main proteins found in the skin and often added to shampoos and conditioners to give "body." Many baldness treatments list it as an ingredient, but no research has established its effectiveness.

COMMON BALDNESS   (See MALE-PATTERN BALDNESS.)

CORTEX   Outer coating of the hair shaft.

CORTISONE   A synthetic hormone derived from the natural steroid hormone, cortisol. Often used to treat allergic reactions, it's also effective against alopecia areata.

CUTICLE   Outer, nonliving coating of the hair, made of protein, which gives hair its sheen and contributes to its strength.

CYSTINE   An amino acid that helps keratin to form in the hair follicle. Keratin is one of the main proteins that makes up the hair shaft.

DANDRUFF   Condition in which the skin constantly replaces itself, with the top two layers changing about once a month. As new cells form, the older ones shed. On the scalp these cells sometimes join to form "flakes" of dandruff. Severe cases could contribute to hair loss, but normal showering and treated shampoos have all but eliminated this condition.

DELAY   A pause or waiting period in a surgical procedure, designed to increase its success. In hair-flap surgery two delays are built into the procedure, so the flap suffers the least amount of trauma and maintains a good blood supply. Thus, it remains very healthy after it is rotated to the top of the bald scalp. (See Chapter 10.)

DERMATITIS   Inflammation of the scalp which creates redness, scaling, and oozing. In severe cases, may cause temporary hair loss.

DERMIS   The "true skin"—located just below the topmost layer or epidermis.

DIABETES   A disease in which the body can't produce or use the insulin necessary to metabolize carbohydrates, including sugar. Skin disorders and hair loss can accompany diabetes.

DIHYDROTESTOSTERONE (DHT)   Derives from the male hormone, testosterone, after the enzyme 5-alpha reductase converts it in the hair follicles. It is a stronger form of testosterone, believed to play a major role in permanent hair loss (baldness).

DONOR AREA   The site from which hair plugs are taken for surgical transplantation into bald scalp. May also refer to the area on the sides and back of the head from which a hair flap is taken.

DONOR DOMINANT   A term first used by Dr. Norman Orentreich, meaning that a punch graft (plug) of skin keeps its own characteristics, no matter where it is transplanted. Makes hair transplants and flap surgery possible.

DOUBLE-BLIND STUDY   Scientific study in which neither the researchers nor the subjects know who receives the test solution and who receives a placebo. Important to hair research because it's the only kind of study that excludes possible bias in observing hair growth. In other words, knowing that a person has received a test solution could otherwise lead researchers to "see" hair growth that doesn't exist.

ECZEMA   A skin disorder that can cause itching, inflammation, or even eruptions with a crusty, scaly residue. In some cases, eczema can lead to temporary hair loss.

ENDROCRINE/ENDOCRINOLOGIST   The endocrine system consists of the glands and tissues that produce the body's hormones. The pituitary gland, pancreas, ovaries, testicles, kidneys, and thyroid are all part of the endocrine system. Endocrinologists are medical doctors who specialize in this area and therefore can treat non-male-pattern baldness resulting from hormone imbalances.

ENZYME   Enzymes are proteins that cause chemical reactions in the body to build cells. The enzyme 5-alpha reductase is particularly important to the study of baldness because it changes testosterone into dihydrotestosterone (DHT), which in turn starts the balding process.

EPIDERMIS   Outer layer of the skin

EPITHELIAL CELLS   The layer of cells forming the epidermis of the skin and the surface thickness of mucous membranes

ESTROGEN   Commonly called female hormones, estradiol and progesterone are both estrogens. The ovaries produce most of a woman's estrogen. In normal men, the adrenal glands develop only a small amount of estrogen. It's possible to reverse male baldness with injections of estrogen but not without side-effects such as enlarged breasts and feminine features.

EUNUCH A castrated male—one whose testicles have been removed. Important to research on balding because eunuchs have no male hormones and never go bald. Thus, reducing the male hormone, testosterone, appears to be directly connected to avoiding hair loss.

FEMALE-PATTERN BALDNESS Common condition in women caused by genes, age, and hormones. Leads to general thinning over the scalp's surface. Occasionally responds to applications of Rogaine (minoxidil) but doesn't lend itself to surgical transplants because it's not confined to distinct areas. Develops much slower than male-pattern baldness and is often not at its height until age 50 or 60.

FIVE (5)-ALPHA REDUCTASE (See 5-ALPHA REDUCTASE under "ALPHA.")

FLAPS/ FLAP GRAFTS A surgical procedure in which a section of the hair-bearing scalp from the side or back of the head is rotated over the top to cover part of a bald area. In most hair-replacement surgery, one end of the flap remains connected to the scalp so it receives its own continuous blood supply. See Chapter 10.

FOLLICLE (See HAIR FOLLICLE.)

FREE GRAFTS Full grafts or strips of hair-bearing scalp that are completely removed from the head and transplanted into bald areas. Unlike flap grafts, they don't have one end attached to the donor area and its blood supply, so they have a very high failure rate.

FRICTION ALOPECIA Hair loss from chronic rubbing as, for example, in hospital patients who lie in one position for a long time.

FUSION (BONDING) A cosmetic solution for baldness in which new hair is woven together in small tufts and then glued or attached with nylon thread to the existing hair.

GENES/GENETIC Each cell in the body carries a strand of "DNA" containing all the information which makes us individuals instead of copies of each other. The information resides in genes that determine such things as our eye color or height. Genes are inherited from the parents. The gene for baldness can come from the mother's or father's side of the family— though it more often seems to trace to the mother's side.

GLYCERIN A syrupy liquid in all animal and vegetable fats and oils which appears to thicken hair when applied to it. Often added to quack baldness treatments but also an ingredient in hair thickeners and other grooming aids.

HAIR ADDITION A hair-replacement unit that covers the bald area on the top and back of the head. Most common method of covering male-pattern baldness.

HAIR BULB Lower, expanded part of a hair root. When cells divide and multiply in an area of the bulb called the matrix, hair forms and grows.

HAIR FOLLICLE A cylindrical depression in the epidermis which houses the hair root and nourishes hair growth.

HAIR PAPILLA "Nipple" of cells that enfold the hair bulb at the bottom of each hair follicle.

HAIRPIECE See HAIR ADDITION.

HAIR ROOT   The part of the hair embedded in the skin at the base of a hair follicle.

HAIR SHAFT   The visible part of the hair—made up of dead protein cells supported by the living cells at the hair root.

HAIR TRANSPLANT   (See TRANSPLANT.)

HORMONES   Hormones develop from the endocrine system and control body functions. They move through the blood stream to genetically determined sites. Although bald men have normal hormone levels, testosterone traveling to the scalp interacts with proteins in the hair follicles to cause baldness in those whose genes are programmed for it.

HEREDITY   Inborn ability of a person to develop characteristics of his or her ancestors. Process by which DNA and genes determine our physical characteristics.

HYPERTENSION   Higher than normal blood pressure. Some drugs that have lowered blood pressure have also grown hair on bald heads (e.g., minoxidil).

HYPERVITAMINOSIS A   Taking in too much Vitamin A, which in severe cases can cause hair loss.

HYPOVITAMINOSIS A   Taking in too little Vitamin A, which can cause temporary hair loss in some cases. Usually a problem only in starvation diets.

IMPLANTS   Placing synthetic hairs directly into the scalp, usually connected to fine wires. Now banned by the Food and Drug Administration because nearly 100 percent of the implants were rejected by the immune systems of those who received them. Many suffered serious and even life-threatening reactions. Transplants, tunnel grafts, and surgically attached hairpieces don't use this technique.

INOSITOL   Deficiencies of this vitamin in lab animals have caused hair loss. Although it's a popular ingredient of many baldness treatments, there's no evidence linking it to male-pattern baldness.

KERATIN   An extremely tough protein substance in hair, nails, and horny tissue.

LANUGO HAIR   Dense, downy growth of early immature hairs. The type of hair covering infants' bodies.

MALE-PATTERN BALDNESS (MPB)   Also called Common Baldness, Pattern Baldness, or Androgenetic Baldness. The most common cause of hair loss in men. MPB is caused by a combination of heredity, male hormone (testosterone), and age. It's distinctive because the hair loss occurs only on the top front and crown of the head. Some hair always remains around the sides and back.

MATRIX   The active, growing part of the hair follicle.

MEDULLA   The inner part of the hair shaft. It gives the shaft its strength and durability.

MELANIN   The pigment which gives color to hair.

MENOPAUSE   Menopause naturally ends a woman's ability to reproduce and may change her hormonal balance between the dominant female hormones and the smaller amounts of male hormones normally present. If a woman has the genetic tendency towards baldness, she may begin to lose hair at this time.

MINIGRAFTS AND MICROGRAFTS   Grafts smaller than the usual three-sixteenths of an inch may be necessary to fill in at the hairline resulting from punch-graft or hair-flap surgery. Minigrafts are about half as large, and even finer effects can be achieved using micrografts (one or two hairs).

MINOXIDIL   A drug made by the Upjohn Company to combat high blood pressure. Marketed as Loniten, it continues to be very effective for this purpose. But a two percent solution of minoxidil has also been marketed since 1988 as a prescription drug for baldness (see ROGAINE).

NIACIN   Nicotinic acid or Vitamin B3. An ingredient in many baldness treatments, despite there being no established connection to male-pattern baldness.

NUTRIENTS   Foods that supply the body with its necessary elements. Usually divided into protein, vitamins, minerals, and so on.

NUTRITION   All the processes by which we take in, absorb, and metabolize food in order for the body to grow, repair itself, or maintain its activities.

PABA   Para-aminobenzoic acid. May help prevent gray hair but has nothing to do with male-pattern baldness.

PANTOTHENIC ACID   A B-complex vitamin that is an important player in cell metabolism. Gray hair may appear when the diet is deficient in pantothenic acid, but it has no apparent effect on male-pattern baldness.

PAPILLA   See HAIR PAPILLA.

PIGMENTED   Having pigmentation or color. Terminal hairs are pigmented whereas the vellus hairs growing on infants and on the scalps of bald people are not.

PLACEBO   A drug substitute that has no chemical effect or action. "Control groups" in scientific studies take a placebo so researchers can more accurately measure the effect of an actual drug given to other patients in the study.

PLUGS   (See PUNCH GRAFTS.)

POLYSORBATE   Polysorbate has been a popular baldness treatment since research from the University of Helsinki in 1978 claimed it could reverse male-pattern baldness. A later study at the University of California didn't back up these claims, but it has still earned millions of dollars for its distributors.

PROGESTERONE   A female hormone that has slowed down or stopped hair loss when injected into the scalps of balding men. Requires a doctor's prescription and may have feminizing effects, such as breast enlargement, soft features, and so on.

PROPYLENE GLYCOL   A liquid chemical often used as a base for baldness formulas or for drugs such as minoxidil.

PUNCH GRAFT   Preferred name for the "plug" of hair and skin taken from a donor area and placed into bald scalp during hair transplantation. Normally circular, about three-sixteenths of an inch in diameter, and containing 10-20 hairs.

PUBERTY   Transitional period of development between childhood and adulthood. Sexual characteristics develop during this period. Males castrated before puberty produce no male hormone (testosterone) and therefore show no signs of balding.

PUVA   One of the treatments for alopecia areata. By coating the bald areas with psoralen, a medication sensitive to light, and then shining ultraviolet light on them, doctors have apparently reversed hair loss. Not effective for male- pattern baldness.

RADIATION   A treatment for cancer that often causes hair loss as a side-effect.

RECEPTOR   A group of cells that receive a stimulus or bond with other cells to form new compounds. Hair follicles have protein receptors that bond with testosterone to form dihydrotestosterone (DHT), which in turn starts the balding process.

RECIPIENT AREA   The bald area that receives hair plugs removed from a donor site during hair-transplant surgery.

REDUCTION   (See SCALP REDUCTION.)

ROGAINE   The brand name given the two percent solution of minoxidil which Upjohn Company markets as an FDA-approved treatment for baldness. More than 300,000 prescriptions were written for Rogaine in 1990, but it appears to have an effectiveness rate of only 10-15 percent for growing some hair on bald crowns.

SCALP REDUCTION   A surgical procedure often used with hair transplants or flap surgery. The surgeon takes out a section of bald scalp about one-half inch wide, usually extending from the middle of the head to the back of the bald spot. He then sutures the sides together, decreasing the bald area and with it the number of transplant plugs needed for full coverage. Used with flap surgery, scalp reduction also stretches the donor area upward and therefore increases the amount of hair available for a flap. See Chapter 8.

SCALP STRETCHING   See TISSUE EXPANSION.

SEBACEOUS GLANDS   Glands in the skin which produce sebum, or oil. Despite claims to the contrary, there is no evidence to connect too much or too little sebum with male-pattern baldness.

SEBORRHEA   Disease of the sebaceous glands which causes them to produce too much oil. In severe cases, may produce Alopecia Seborrheica, a usually temporary hair loss that is not connected to male-pattern baldness.

SEBUM   (See SEBACEOUS GLANDS.)

STRIP GRAFTS   (See FREE GRAFTS.)

TAGAMET   Another name for an ulcer drug, cimetidine, made by Smith, Kline, and French. Presently under testing to determine whether it can slow down hair loss.

TELOGEN   One of the three phases of hair growth, usually called the resting stage. In this stage the follicle is resting and no hair is visible. The previous hair has fallen out, and a new hair will start growing with the next anagen (growth) phase. About 10 percent of our hairs are in telogen at any given time.

TELOGEN EFFLUVIUM   Usually temporary hair loss that follows any kind of stress, such as a fever, surgical operation, childbirth, or emotional disturbance. Occurs after transplant surgery and thus delays hair growth by several months. Doesn't occur in flap surgery, probably because the flap has its own blood supply through the temporal artery.

TERMINAL HAIRS   Normal, adult hairs which contrast with the fine, usually uncolored vellus hairs on new-born babies and the scalps of bald men. Baldness treatments that claim to grow hair may be talking about vellus hairs, which have little cosmetic effect on baldness.

TESTOSTERONE   The most powerful male hormone. If a man has a genetic tendency to baldness, he may go bald with a normal level of testosterone. Women also produce a very small amount of testosterone, but this level can increase after menopause and produce hair loss for some women.

TOPICAL   Applied to the surface and affecting only that part of the body. If a substance affects the entire body, such as a pill or a liquid to be swallowed, it has a systemic rather than a topical effect.

TOUPEE   (See HAIR ADDITION.)

TRACTION ALOPECIA   Hair loss from a constant pulling on the hair by tight braids, ponytails, hair weaving, and some methods of attaching hairpieces. Any steady pressure on the hair can cause permanent thinning spots if maintained too long.

TRICHOTILLOMANIA   The unnatural compulsion to pull out one's own hair. Usually found only in children and young adults and typically caused by an emotional disturbance.

TUNNEL GRAFTS   A surgical method of attaching a hairpiece. The surgeon creates little loops of skin and sutures them into the bald scalp. Matching ties and clips on the hairpiece firmly attach to these tunnel skin grafts and hold the hairpiece in place.

VELLUS HAIRS   Very fine, uncolored hair on newborn babies and the scalps of bald men.

VERTEX   Top of the head, or crown.

WEAVING   A way to attach a hairpiece using a bald man's natural hair as an anchor. A stylist may weave the base of an entire hairpiece into a braided fringe of hair around the bald area. An alternate method is to weave additional hair through a mesh attached to the fringe hair and any other hair that a balding man may have left. Weaving holds a hairpiece firmly but may cause hair loss because of traction. It also loosens up as natural hair grows out, so it needs frequent tightening at a salon.

WIG   A hairpiece that covers the entire scalp, including the sides and back. Less likely to be used for male-pattern baldness than the toupee (hairpiece), but useful for total baldness resulting from burns, disease, or cancer therapy.

Avila, Eva. *The Art of Making Hairpieces for Men*. Las Vegas, Nevada: Blue Diamond Publishing Company, 1991.

Anderson, John. "Interview on Techniques and Materials for Non-Surgical Hair Additions." Colorado Springs, Colorado: V.I.P. Hair Center, Inc, November 18, 1992.

Baden, Howard. *Diseases of the Hair and Nails*. New York: Year Book Medical Publishers, 1987.

Baum, Eileen. "Thin, Thinning, Gone." *Health* 21 (January 1989): 74-76.

Bower, B. "Proteins Point to Roots of Baldness." *Science News* 133 (May 14, 1988): 311.

Brodin, Michael B. "Drug-Related Alopecia." *Dermatologic Clinics* 5,3 (1987): 571-579.

Cannell, David W. "Permanent Waving and Hair Straightening." *Clinics in Dermatology* 6,3 (July-September 1988): 71-82.

___. "Through the Microscope: The Chemistry and Physiology of Human Hair." Redken Laboratories, Inc.: Canoga Park, CA, 1991.

Cash, Thomas F. "Losing Hair, Losing Points?: The Effects of Male Pattern Baldness on Social Impression Formation." *Journal of Applied Social Psychology* 20,2(1990):154-167.

___. "The Psychological Effects of Androgenetic Alopecia in Men." *Journal of the American Academy of Dermatology* 26(1992):926-931.

Dillard-Rosen, Sandra. "Hair: New Look for the '90s," *Denver Post* (January 7, 1990), Contemporary section, p. 10.

Ebling, F. John G. "The Biology of Hair." *Dermatologic Clinics* 5,3 (1987): 467-481.

Ferriman, David G. *Human Hair Growth in Health and Disease*. Springfield: Charles C. Thomas, 1971.

Flynn, Suzanne K. *How to Save Your Hair*. New York: Arbor House, 1984.

Gale, Bill. *The Mature Man's Guide to Style*. New York: William Morrow and Company, Inc., 1980.

Haberman, Fredric and Margaret Danbrot. *The Doctor's Beauty Hotline*. New York: Henry Holt and Company, Inc., 1990.

Inkeles, Stephen B., William E. Connor, and D. Roger Illingworth. "Hepatic and Dermatologic Manifestations of Chronic Hypervitaminosis A in Adults." *American Journal of Medicine* 80 (1986): 491-496.

Kaufman, J. P. "Telogen Effluvium Secondary to Starvation Diet." *Archives of Dermatology* 112 (1976): 731.

Korbori, Tatsuji and William Montagna, eds. *Biology and Disease of the Hair*. Baltimore: University Park Press, 1976.

Lippert, J.L. "Hair, Glorious Hair," *Health* 19 (May 1987): 58-60+.

REFERENCES

Lucky, Anne W. "The Paradox of Balding: Where Are We Now?" *Journal of Investigative Dermatology* 91,2 (1988): 99-100.

Mayer, Toby G. and Richard W. Fleming. *Aesthetic and Reconstructive Surgery of the Scalp.* St. Louis, MO: Mosby-Year Book, Inc., 1992.

Michael, George and Rae Lindsay. *George Michael's Complete Hair Care for Men.* Garden City, NY: Doubleday, 1983.

Mitchell, Andrew J. and Mark R. Balle. "Alopecia Areata." *Dermatologic Clinics* 5,3 (1987): 553-564.

Mizel, Steven B., M.D. and Peter Jaret. *In Self Defense: The Human Immune System.* New York: Harcourt Brace, 1985.

Orentreich, Norman and R. Rizer. *Medical Treatment of Androgenetic Alopecia.* New York: Praeger, 1980.

Pervan, Anthony S. *Natural Hair Growth.* Hollywood, FL: Fell, 1987.

Sadick, Neil S. and Donald C. Richardson. *Your Hair: Helping to Keep It.* Yonkers, NY: Consumers Union of the United States, Inc., 1991.

Saffon, M. J. with Charles Francisco. *Complete Skin and Hair Care Program for the Active Man.* Piscataway, NJ: New Century Publishers, Inc., 1986.

Schoen, Linda, ed. *The AMA Book of Skin and Hair Care.* New York: Avon, 1984.

___ and Paul Lazar. *The Look You Like: Medical Answers to 400 Questions on Skin and Hair Care.* New York: Marcel Dekker, Inc., 1990.

Spencer, Linda V. and Jeffrey P. Callen. "Hair Loss in Systemic Disease." *Dermatologic Clinics* 5,3 (1987): 565-570.

Woodruff, David. "For Rogaine, No Miracle Cure--Yet," *Business Week* (June 4, 1990): 100.

A

Age
hair loss and. *See* Hair loss: age-related
Alopecia areata   15–16
Alopecia seborrheica   13
Anagen   13–14
Androgenetic alopecia. *See* Male-pattern baldness
Anti-androgens   82–83
Axial flaps   159–160

B

Bald crown
styling for   37–38
Baldness "treatments"   67–78
Biotin   75–76
Blood flow
increasing to cure baldness   71–74
Bonding. *See* Hair bonding
Brushing   29–30

C

Cabling. *See* Hair weaving
Cash, Thomas   7, 85
Catagen   13–14
Chemotherapy
temporary hair loss and   16–17
Class III baldness. *See* Male-pattern baldness
Combing   29–30
Combs   42
Conditioning   31
Cortex   12
Cortisone   16
Cyoctol   82–83

D

Dandruff   17–18
Delay   122
Diazoxide   85–86
Diets   18
Dihydrotestosterone (DHT)   28, 76
Doctors
choosing   173
Donor dominance   102
Drugs
temporary hair loss and   16–17

E

Electrical devices
as baldness cures   73–74

F

Female-pattern hair loss. *See* Hair loss: females
Flap surgery   121
crown baldness and   135–136
delay   122, 123–124
for a second flap   128–129
hairstyling after   137
history of   121–122
micrografts and   133
post-surgical care   124, 125–126
procedure   123–125
scalp reductions and   129–131
Follicle. *See* Hair Follicle
Forehead lift   141
post-surgical care   146–147
procedure for men   145
procedure for women   144
results of   147–148
Free flaps   162
disadvantages of   162
Fusion   56–57

G

Galea   71–72
Galeal thinners
as a baldness cure   72–73
Grooming aids   32

H

Hair additions   43–66
custom-made   46
disadvantages   65–66
errors in using   60
foundations   46–47
getting a natural look   57–58
hair coloring and   50
hair texture and   50
hairlines and   48–50
methods of attachment   51–56
ready-made   45–46
surgery and   64

ventilation technique   48

Hair analysis   76–78

Hair bonding   61–62

Hair coloring   34

Hair curling
    and hair damage   32

Hair damage   30–32

Hair devices
    hair loss and   19

Hair flap
    description of   121

Hair follicle   11–13, 14
    unclogging as a baldness cure   68–71

Hair growth   11

Hair growth cycle   13–14

Hair implants
    dangers of   62–63

Hair integration   59–61

Hair loss
    age-related   23–24
    females and   24–25
    heredity and   28
    hormones and   24
    permanent   23
    physical injury and   23
    temporary   15

Hair popping   73

Hair shedding   13–14

Hair straightening
    and hair damage   32

Hair structure   11

Hair transplants   101
    age and   103–104
    cobblestoning   114–115
    complications   114–115
    cost of   119
    disadvantages   120
    donor hair and   105–107
    hair color and   107
    hair texture and   102–103
    hairstyling and   118
    limitations   101
    micrografts   115–116
    minigrafts   115–116
    post-surgical care   113

procedure   102–103, 110–112

Hair weaving   56

Hairline
    in hair-replacement surgery   107–109

Hairstyling   29–42
    facial features and   32–33
    styles to avoid   41
    thinning hair and   34–35

Human hair
    in hair additions   43–45

Hypothyroidism   21

I

Immune system research   86–87

Incisional slit grafting   117

Infection
    temporary hair loss and   21

J

Juri, Jose   122

K

Keratin   11–12, 14

L

Lamont, E.S.   122

M

Male-pattern baldness   25–28. *See also* Hair loss
    classifications   26–27
    myths about   28
    styling for   38–39

Medulla   12

Micrografts   115–116

Minigrafts   115–116

Minoxidil   67, 79–80

N

Nutriol   75

Nutrition
    as a baldness cure   74–78
    temporary hair loss and   18–19

P

Papilla   11–12

Passot, Raymond   121–122

Patchy baldness. *See* Alopecia areata
Permanent waving   39–41
Polysorbate   69–71
Pregnancy
    hair shedding and   14
Prescription drugs to cure baldness   79
Pressure alopecia   19–20
Progesterone   81–82
Proscar   86
Protein   18
Psoriasis   17–18
Punch grafting. *See* Hair transplants

R

Random flaps   160–162
    disadvantages of   160–161
Razor cutting   42
Receding hairline
    styling for   36–37
Reconstructive surgery   163
Rogaine. *See* Minoxidil

S

Scalp elasticity   97
Scalp massage   72
Scalp reductions   89
    complications   94
    cosmetic problems after   95
    the Marzola procedure   97–100
    patterns for   90–92
    procedure for   92–94
    when to avoid   97
Sebaceous glands   13
    poor nutrition and   18–19
    seborrhea and   17
Seborrhea   17–18
Sebum   13, 18
    excess as cause of baldness   68
Shampooing   30
Shedding. *See* Hair shedding
Short flaps   157–159
    design of   157–158
    procedure for   158
    uses for   158–159
Styling. *See* Hairstyling

Synthetic hair
    in hair additions   43–45

T

Telogen   13–14
Telogen effluvium   20–21
    extensive scalp reductions and   99
Terminal hair   13
Testosterone   25, 81–83
Thinning hair. *See* Hairstyling: thinning hair
Tissue expansion   149
    advantages of   153–155
    complications from   153
    disadvantages of   155–156
    procedure for   150–151
    questions about   151–152
    types of expanders   150
Toupee. *See* Hair additions
Traction alopecia   19
Transplants. *See* Hair transplants
Trichotillomania   19
Tricomin   86

V

Vasodilation   72
Vellus hair   13
Viprostol   84–85
Vitamin A   18–19
Vitamins
    hair growth and   74

W

Weaving. *See* Hair weaving
Wigs   64

Acknowledgments

We wish to thank all who have contributed to the quality and content of this book, but a few people deserve special mention. Michael Mahoney and John Anderson reviewed our information regarding hair additions and shared their expertise on fabrication procedures, selection of hair types, and fastening methods. Don McCoy added pertinent comments on hair styling and permanent waving for men with thinning hair. Adamo Lentini's professional styling helped illustrate our discussion on proper styling techniques for thinning hair in Chapter Four. Irene Luckett's meticulous research and Perry Luckett's careful editing of the entire book helped make our work more accurate and complete. Finally, we gratefully acknowledge the efforts of Rob Feinberg, who—as designer and publisher— shepherded The Everyman's Guide to Hair Replacement through nearly three years of research and writing to arrive at its present form.

Photographs are courtesy of The Beverly Hills Institute of Aesthetic and Reconstructive Surgery except for those in Chapter 5, "Non-Surgical Hair Additions," which are courtesy of Michael Mahoney. Illustrations are by Timothy C. Hengst, except for figures 6-1 and 6-2, which are courtesy of the Bettmann Archives.